STROKE RECOVERY

Activity Book

Name: _ _ _ _ _ _ _ _ _ _ _ _ _ _ _ _ _ _ _

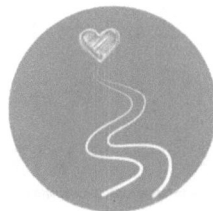

**Vital Steps
Books**

Welcome to your **Stroke Recovery Activity Book**. We deeply appreciate your trust in choosing our resource to aid your journey towards recovery. This book is thoughtfully divided into sections, each designed to strengthen different essential skills for your rehabilitation.

Within these sections, you will find validated activities of varied levels, allowing you to progress at your own pace and challenge yourself as you regain and enhance your capabilities. **Thank you** for allowing us to be a part of your recovery. We are here to support you every step of the way.

Follow us:

www.vitalstepsbooks.com

INDEX

Cognitive Skills

-Attention and Concentration

-Chronological Events

-Word Association

★ **Usefulness:**

Memory Improvement
Enhanced Concentration
Sharper Problem-Solving
Stronger Executive Functions

INSTRUCTIONS

📌 It is advised not to use a highlighter as it could bleed through the page.

📌 In some statements, the explanation of the exercise is highlighted. In these cases, it involves an additional task to be performed to increase the difficulty of the exercise.

📌 The solutions are found at the end of each section.

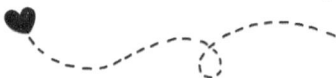

Outsider - 1

Find the exception. Examine the grid, one shape is not like the others. Circle that shape.

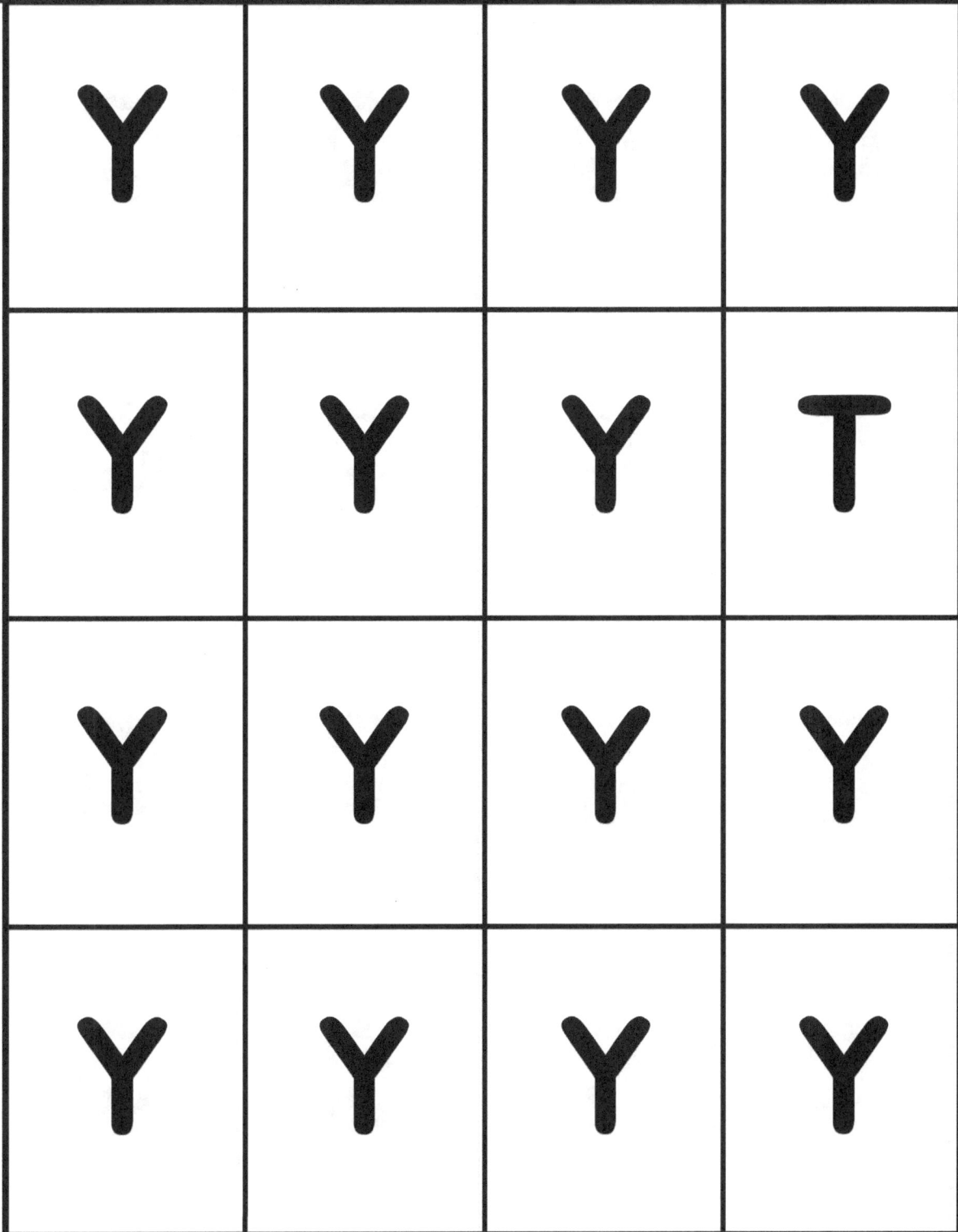

Y	Y	Y	Y
Y	Y	Y	T
Y	Y	Y	Y
Y	Y	Y	Y

Outsider - 2

Find the exception. Examine the grid, one shape is not like the others. Circle that shape.

Q	Q	Q	Q
Q	Q	Q	Q
Q	Q	Q	O
Q	Q	Q	Q

Outsider - 3

Find the exception. Examine the grid, one shape is not like the others. Circle that shape.

b	b	b	b	b
b	b	b	b	b
b	b	b	d	b
b	b	b	b	b
b	b	b	b	b

Outsider - 4

j	j	j	j	j
j	j	j	j	j
j	j	j	j	i
j	j	j	j	j
j	j	j	j	j

8

Outsider - 5

Find the exception. Examine the grid, one shape is not like the others. Circle that shape.

W	W	W	W	W
W	W	W	W	W
W	W	W	W	W
W	W	W	W	W
W	W	V	W	W
W	W	W	W	W

Outsider - 6

Find the exception. Examine the grid, one shape is not like the others. Circle that shape.

6	6	6	6	6	6	6
6	6	6	6	6	6	6
6	6	6	6	6	6	6
6	6	6	6	6	6	6
6	9	6	6	6	6	6
6	6	6	6	6	6	6
6	6	6	6	6	6	6
6	6	6	6	6	6	6

Before and after

Write the numbers that come before and after the middle number. There is an example in the box.

8	9	10

f) ☐ 7 ☐

a) ☐ 6 ☐

g) ☐ 11 ☐

b) ☐ 3 ☐

h) ☐ 3 ☐

c) ☐ 5 ☐

i) ☐ 8 ☐

d) ☐ 12 ☐

j) ☐ 4 ☐

e) ☐ 18 ☐

k) ☐ 2 ☐

Lost Dots

Complete the addition so that the result equals the number on the right. You may write the number or draw the dots.

a) [⚁] + [ ] = 6

b) [ ] + [⚃] = 8

c) [⚀] + [ ] = 4

d) [ ] + [⚁] = 3

e) [⚀] + [ ] = 3

f) [⚃] + [ ] = 5

g) [ ] + [⚅] = 7

h) [⚂] + [ ] = 6

i) [ ] + [⚄] = 8

j) [⚃] + [ ] = 9

On the Beach

Look at the pictures below and find the differences.

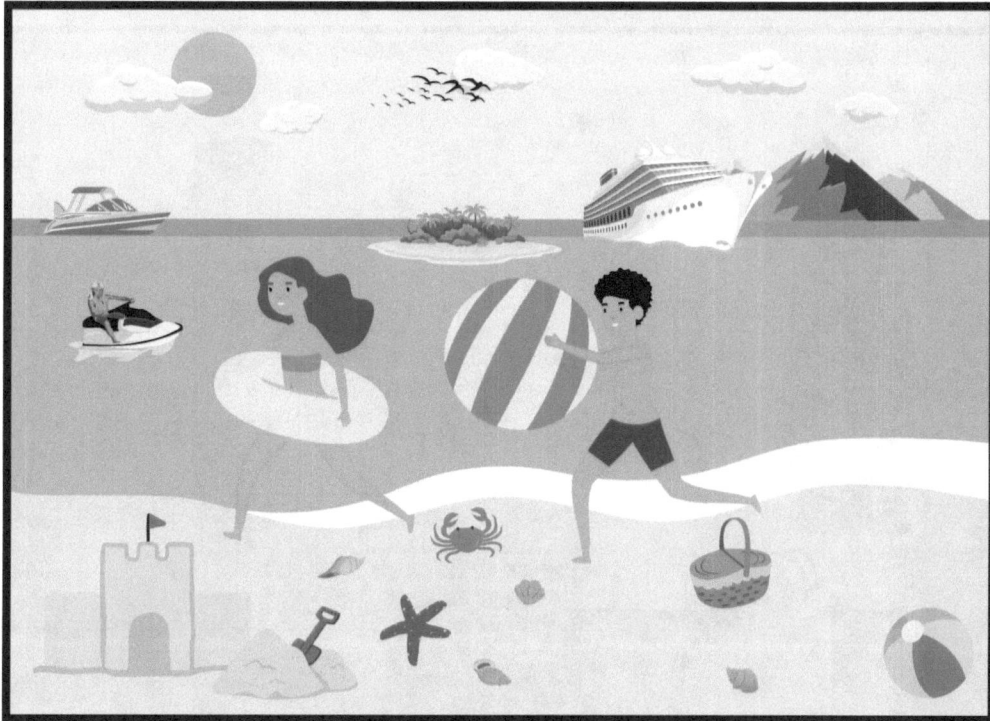

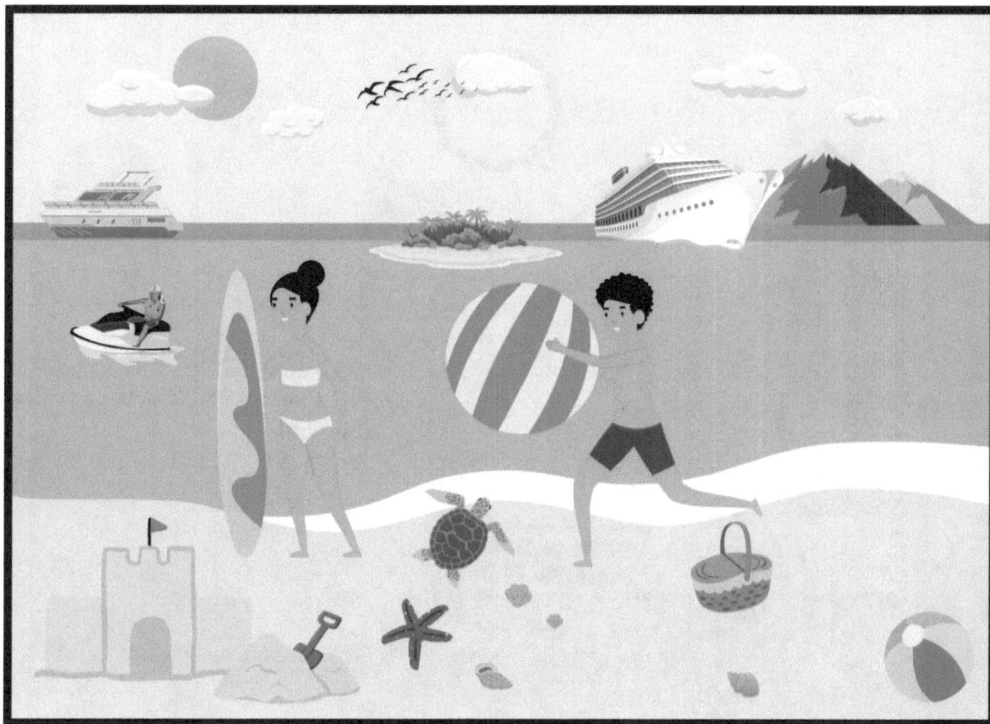

Shopping

Look at the pictures below and find the differences.

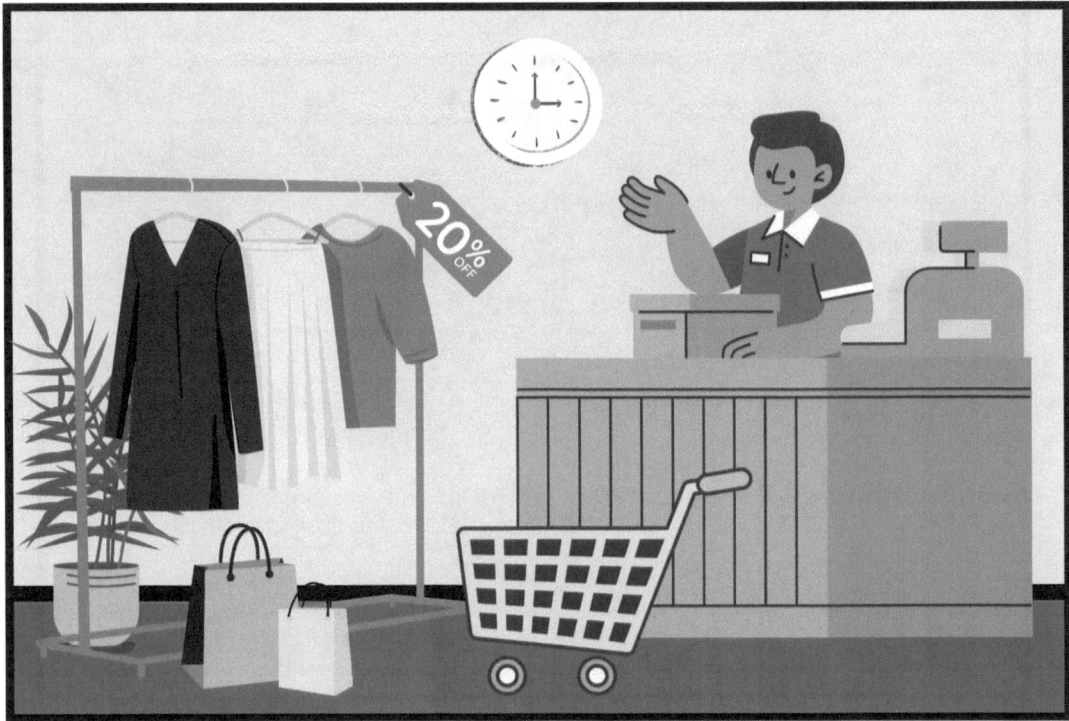

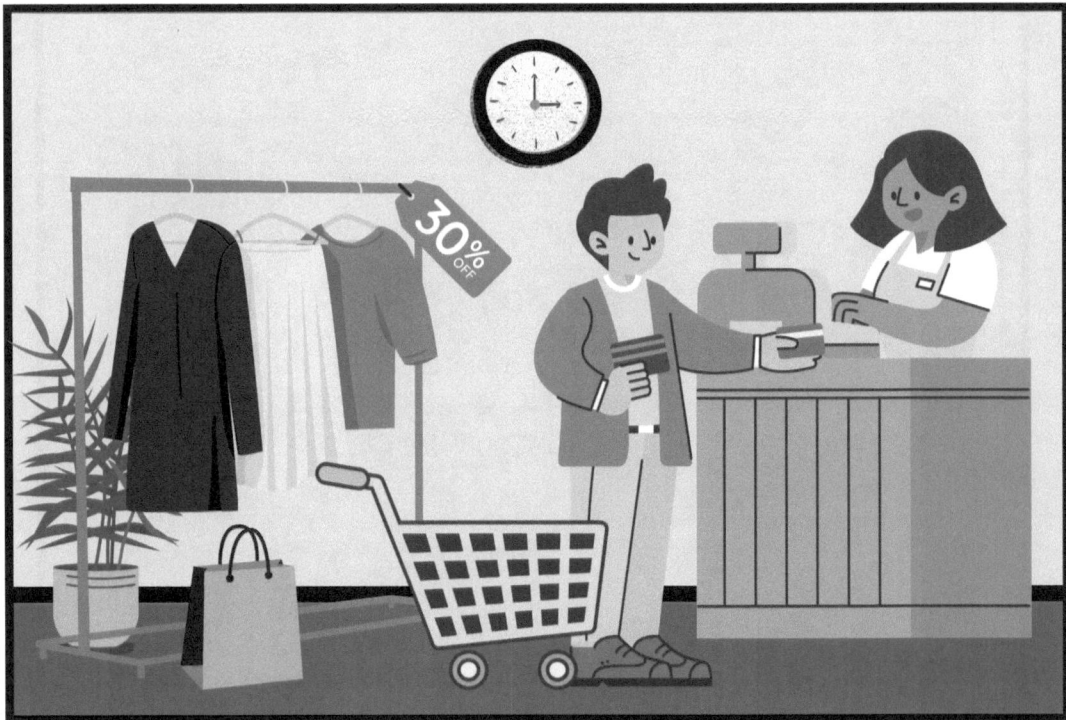

Word Search - 1

Find in the grid the words from the box below. Words can be just vertical or horizontal.

J	W	O	H	T	G	K	S	O	I	E	N
Y	E	Z	F	P	D	S	T	A	N	D	W
B	Q	K	H	D	T	E	R	D	G	F	C
N	B	A	L	A	N	C	E	Z	W	L	N
E	F	W	A	O	A	Z	T	P	P	Q	Y
O	W	J	G	A	J	G	C	N	F	S	J
Z	A	R	R	E	A	C	H	T	O	H	J
D	L	N	I	A	U	U	G	K	C	A	C
B	K	K	P	K	L	W	O	Q	V	H	J
I	S	E	C	K	Z	F	T	L	H	P	V
M	P	I	L	R	N	Q	P	T	A	J	N
B	Y	X	X	D	B	W	T	W	U	Z	V

GRIP	WALK	STAND
REACH	BALANCE	STRETCH

15

Word Search - 2

Find in the grid the words from the box below. Words can be just vertical or horizontal.

S	K	S	I	W	D	O	S	D	P	B	B	E
P	R	E	M	E	M	B	E	R	N	N	E	G
E	E	M	V	R	S	C	T	H	O	Q	W	Y
A	C	U	L	H	X	Y	A	E	I	U	L	G
K	A	L	O	M	C	W	C	G	Q	H	I	B
Y	L	P	U	W	R	U	M	N	R	Q	S	P
P	L	I	X	W	R	I	T	E	H	D	T	P
K	Z	M	D	R	R	E	A	D	E	K	E	Z
C	M	S	Q	H	T	X	A	G	B	T	N	B
O	X	Z	W	Z	W	N	I	R	N	D	C	I
F	G	D	K	R	K	T	C	M	M	F	Y	Z
I	U	D	F	H	Y	N	P	I	D	B	F	I
P	Z	N	S	W	F	D	F	Q	W	L	R	B

READ	SPEAK	WRITE
LISTEN	RECALL	REMEMBER

16

Word Search - 3

Find in the grid the words from the box below. Words can be just vertical or horizontal.

C	M	S	I	B	E	G	Q	A	I	S	S
D	B	M	Q	Z	E	U	B	H	Q	P	Z
A	B	D	K	M	Q	P	S	T	R	J	U
V	B	R	M	U	Z	C	M	A	G	U	K
C	A	G	R	B	Y	E	M	W	H	H	B
A	D	P	R	R	A	O	J	X	I	L	I
L	G	F	E	E	L	V	X	N	D	C	K
M	S	N	S	A	W	C	S	G	F	B	G
H	E	C	T	T	N	N	L	Z	I	H	B
D	C	S	T	H	U	R	E	L	A	X	Q
Y	W	J	K	E	A	I	E	M	D	O	Y
E	W	E	J	R	H	I	P	L	T	S	L

FEEL	REST	CALM
RELAX	SLEEP	BREATHE

17

Word Search - 4

Find in the grid the words from the box below. Words can be just vertical or horizontal.

R	C	L	Z	P	D	T	Y	R	L	G	X	C
A	W	C	E	N	D	H	E	N	T	M	G	G
B	P	T	L	K	O	R	D	B	H	U	K	C
K	P	E	I	G	J	R	W	D	F	T	P	I
Q	R	T	B	M	J	M	H	T	W	F	L	D
R	A	V	X	O	F	W	B	A	E	Z	A	Z
G	C	B	C	W	J	H	G	U	O	N	N	K
T	T	L	M	Q	K	A	D	S	S	P	K	H
F	I	Y	H	T	H	I	N	K	O	O	I	O
N	C	L	Z	L	W	X	I	T	L	Q	U	R
L	E	A	R	N	W	I	A	L	V	I	A	V
I	O	B	D	C	H	O	O	S	E	I	A	Z
B	V	F	N	U	Z	T	R	X	M	K	G	W

PLAN	THINK	SOLVE
LEARN	CHOOSE	PRACTICE

Egg Sequence

Observe the pictures and arrange them according to the sequence order.

a)

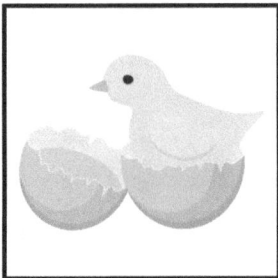

b)

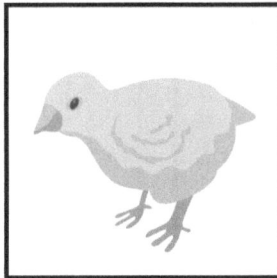

c)

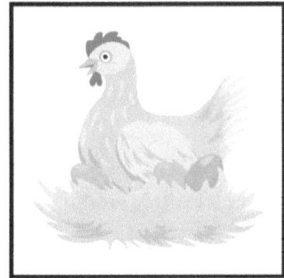

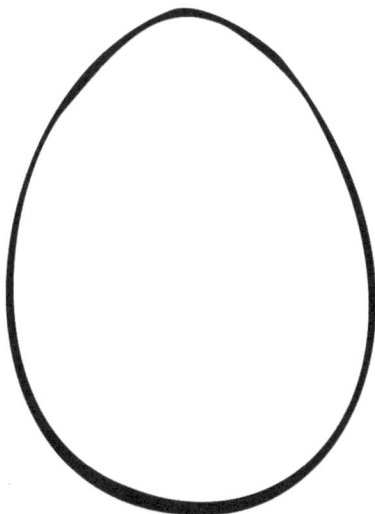

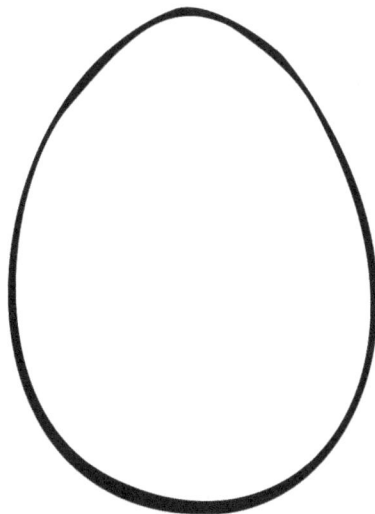

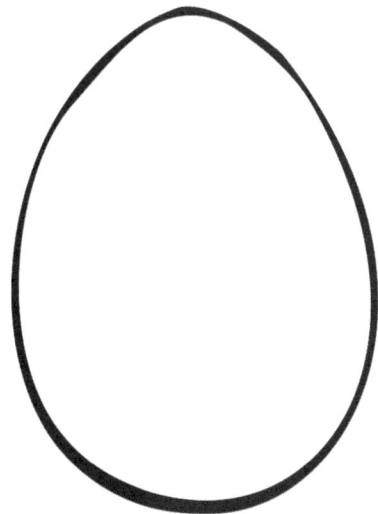

First   Next   Last

Sunflower Sequence

Observe the pictures and arrange them according to the sequence order.

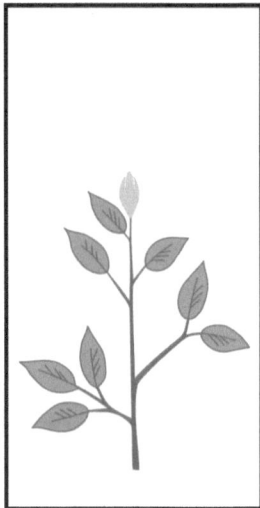 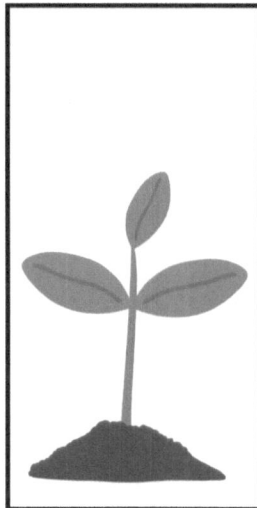 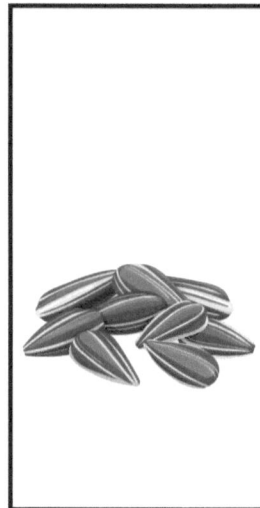 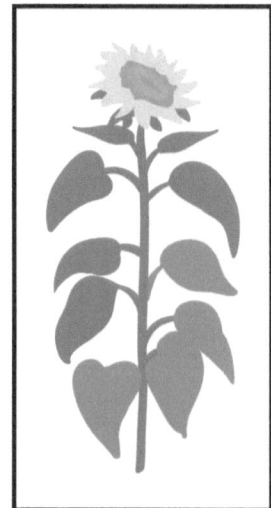

a)   b)   c)   d)

Daily Routine

Think about your daily routine and order the following images according to how you perform them.

REHABILITATION EXERCISES →

SLEEP →

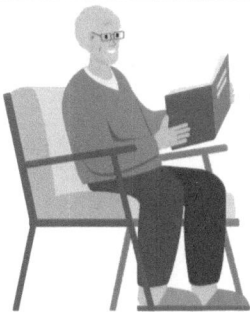

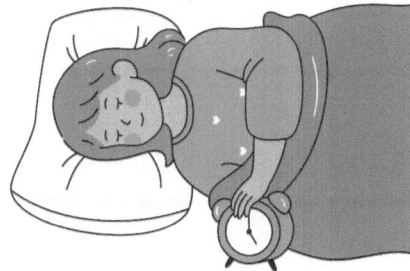

BREAKFAST →

WAKE UP →

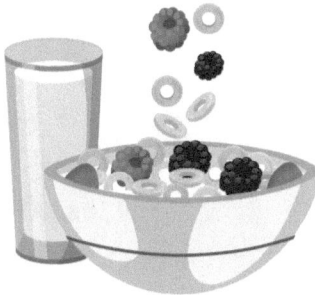

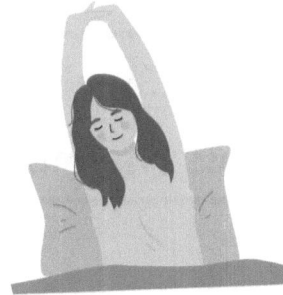

DINNER →

BATH →

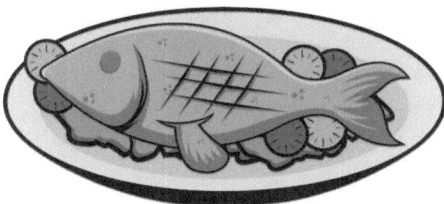

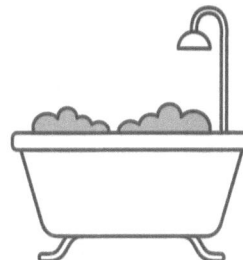

Routine 1: Getting Ready for Bed

Read the boxes and arrange them according to the sequence order. You can use the pictures for assistance.

Turn off lights and other electronics in the house → [ ]

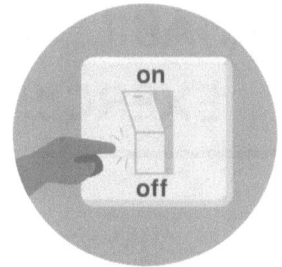

Change into pajamas → [ ]

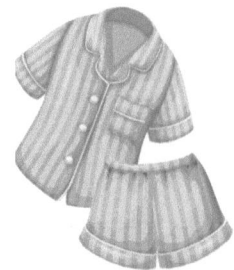

Get into bed and set the alarm for the morning → [ ]

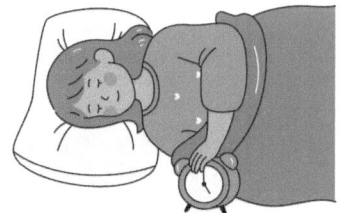

Use the bathroom to brush your teeth and wash your face → [ ]

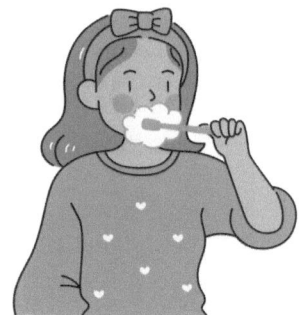

Routing 2: Preparing to Go to the Grocery Store

Read the boxes and arrange them according to the sequence order. You can use the pictures for assistance.

Lock the door behind you as you leave the house → [ ]

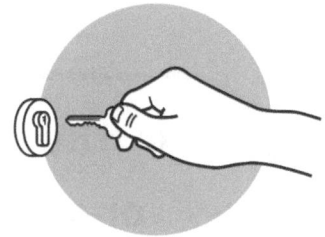

Grab reusable shopping bags and the list → [ ]

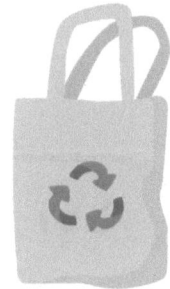

Write a shopping list of needed items → [ ]

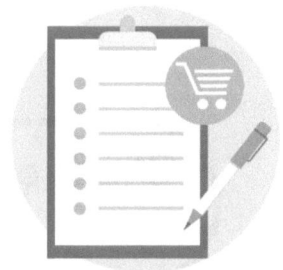

Put on a coat and shoes → [ ]

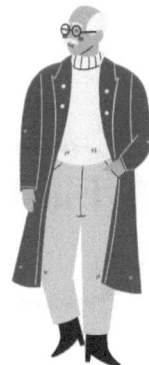

Routine 3: Making a cup of tea

Read the boxes and arrange them according to the sequence order. You can use the pictures for assistance.

Pour the hot water into the cup once the kettle is boiling → [ ]

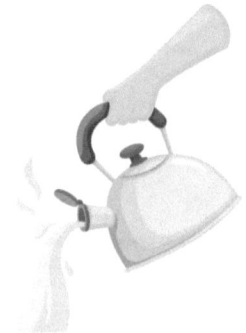

Let the tea steep for a few minutes before drinking → [ ]

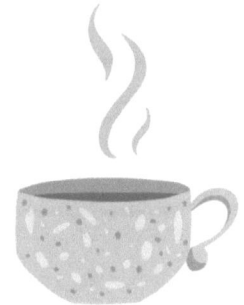

Choose a teabag and place it in the cup → [ ]

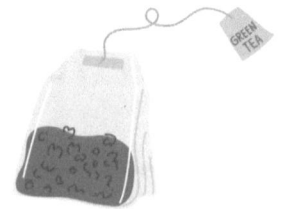

Fill the kettle with water and turn it on → [ ]

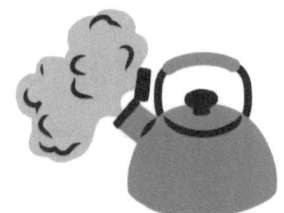

Routine 4: Watching a Favorite TV Show

Read the boxes and arrange them according to the sequence order. You can use the pictures for assistance.

Find the show in the TV guide and watch it at the scheduled time → [ ]

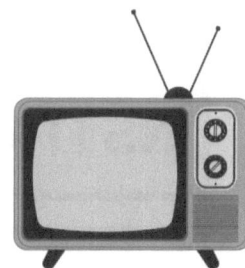

Turn on the television and select the correct channel → [ ]

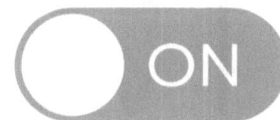

Sit down on a comfortable chair or sofa → [ ]

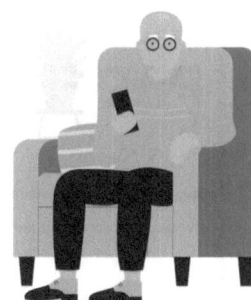

Use the remote to set the volume to a comfortable level → [ ]

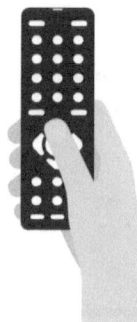

Matching - 1

Connect the words from the column on the right with the categories they belong to on the left.

Try to pronounce the words.

MUSICAL INSTRUMENTS	HAMMER
FURNITURE	BICYCLE
VEHICLES	GUITAR
PROFESSIONS	PASTA
TOOLS	DOCTOR
FOODS	CHAIR

Matching - 1

Connect the words from the column on the right with the categories they belong to on the left.

Try to pronounce the words.

FLOWERS	APPLE
SPORTS	TV
FRUITS	CAT
APPLIANCES	TENNIS
CLOTHING	ROSE
ANIMALS	SHIRT

Matching - 3

Connect the pictures from the column on the right with the categories they belong to on the left.
Try to describe the images.

BEACH

SCHOOL

KITCHEN

WEATHER

BODY PARTS

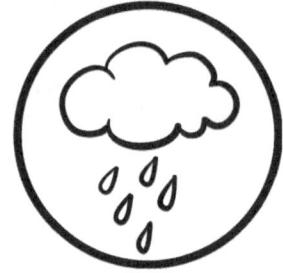

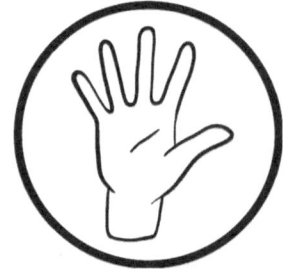

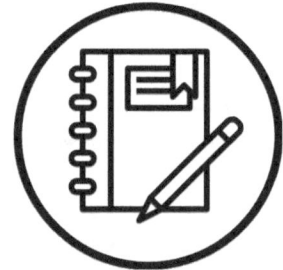

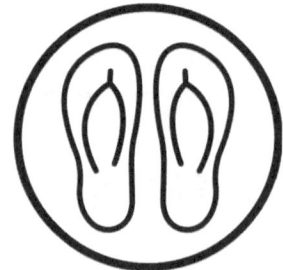

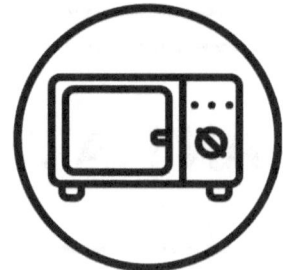

Fruits

Observe the images on the grid and circle those that belong to the fruit category.
<u>Try to describe what the category of the other images would be.</u>

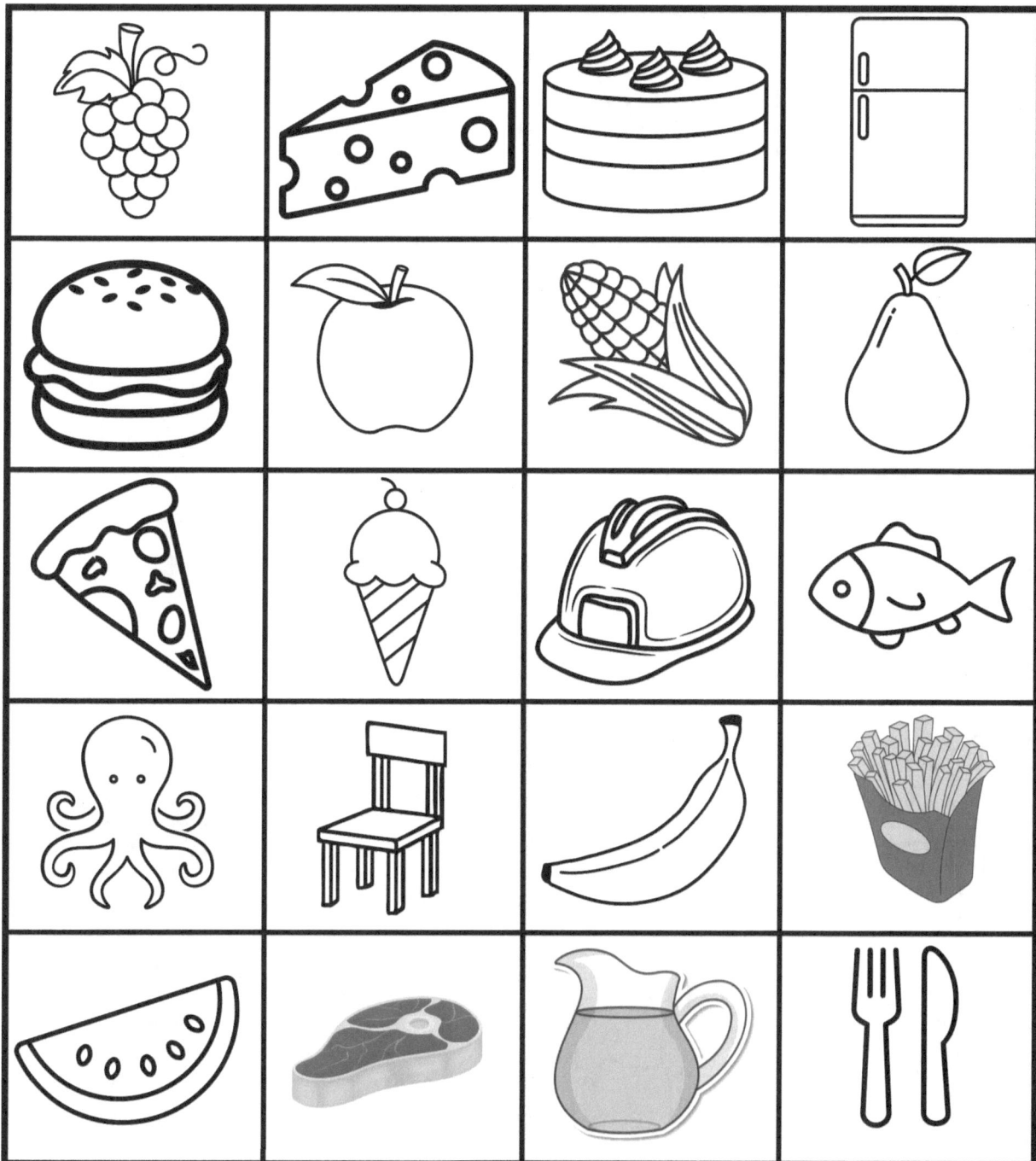

Animals

Observe the images on the grid and circle those that belong to the animals category.
<u>Try to describe what the category of the other images would be.</u>

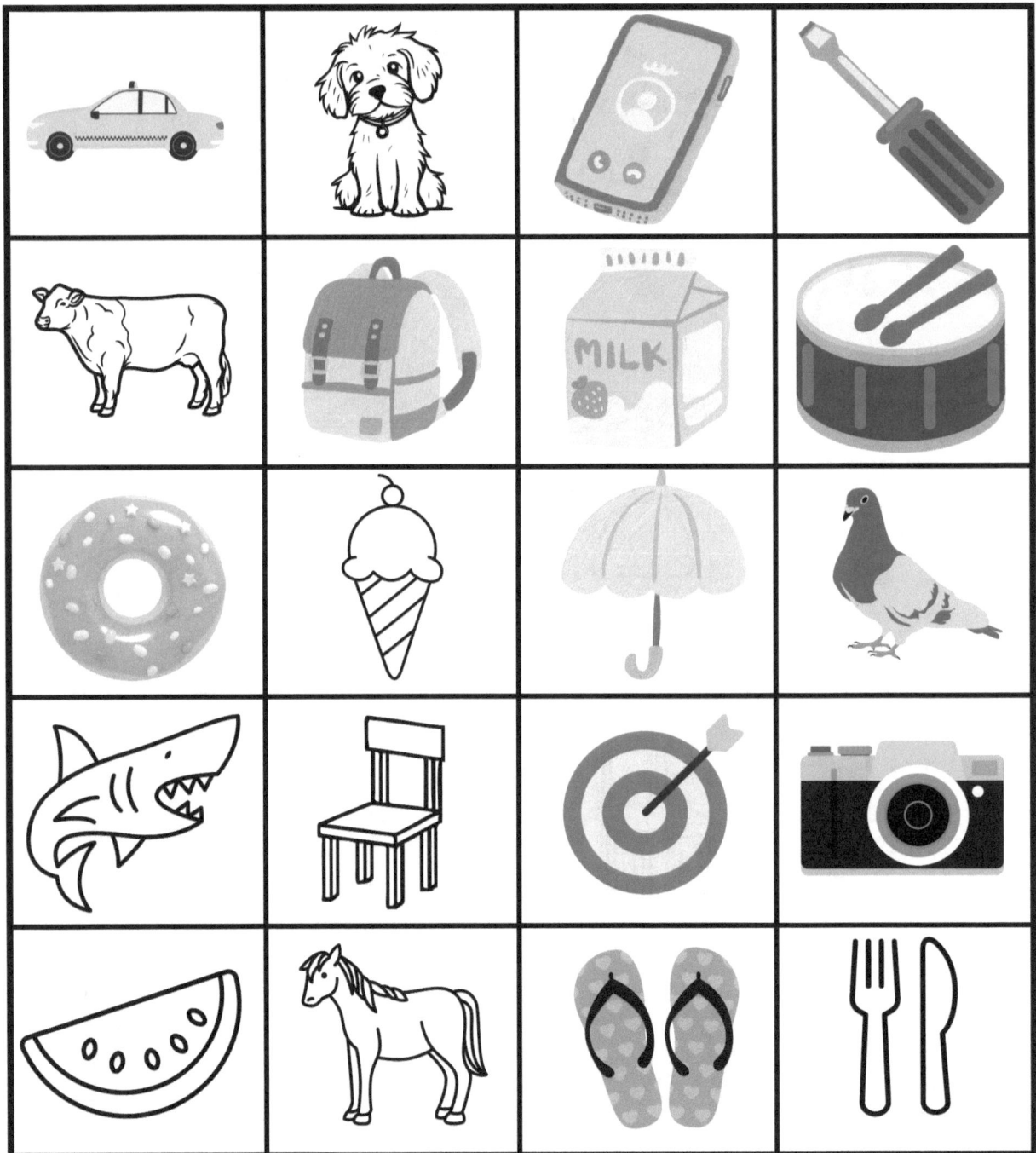

Family

Observe the words on the grid and circle those that belong to the family category.
Try to imagine each word.

CARD	GRANDSON	OVEN	DOCTOR
HEATING	COFFEE	DAUGHTER	PIZZA
DOOR	MOTHER	CUP	GARDEN
UNCLE	PHONE	PEN	FLOOR
TAXI	HOSPITAL	WIFE	BOTTLE

Synonyms

Match the words from the left column with their synonym on the right.

HAPPY	LARGE
SAD	QUICK
BIG	TINY
SMALL	CHILLY
FAST	JOYFUL
SLOW	DIFFICULT
HOT	SIMPLE
COLD	WARM
EASY	UNHAPPY
HARD	SLUGGISH

Antonyms

Match the words from the left column with their antonym on the right.

OLD	POOR
TALL	DRY
RICH	DUMB
SMART	NEW
FULL	FAR
GOOD	UGLY
PRETTY	SHORT
WET	BAD
NEAR	LOW
HIGH	EMPTY

Word Association - 1

Match the words in the left column with those that best match them in the right column.

SUN	SKY
MOON	SAND
STARS	LEAVES
OCEAN	LIGHT
BEACH	BED
FLOWER	GARDEN
TREE	NIGHT
SLEEP	WAVES

Word Association - 2

Match the words in the left column with those that best match them in the right column.

COFFEE	CALL
TEA	LOCK
MEAL	MORNING
GLASSES	MAIL
COMPUTER	AFTERNOON
PHONE	TECHNOLOGY
LETTER	RESTAURANT
KEY	VISION

Connection - 1

Connect each digit with its word.
<u>Try to pronounce the words.</u>

0	THREE
3	NINETEEN
5	SEVENTEEN
8	TWELVE
12	FIVE
17	TWENTY-THREE
19	ZERO
23	EIGHT

Connection - 2

Connect each digit with its word.
Try to pronounce the words.

1	FOUR
4	THIRTEEN
6	FIFTEEN
9	ONE
13	SIX
15	TWENTY-TWO
18	NINE
22	EIGHTEEN

Categories

Write up to six words related to each category.
You can do it at different times.

Vehicles: . . . .

. . . .

Colors: . . . .

. . . .

Tools: . . . .

. . . .

Foods: . . . .

. . . .

Carry On

Write two words related to each category.
You can do it at different times.

Cat - Tiger - .... - ....

Rabbit - Tulip - .... - ....

Parrot - Table - .... - ....

Elephant - Tiger - .... - ....

Tea - Apple - .... - ....

Egg - Grape - .... - ....

Eagle - Elevator - .... - ....

Tree - Elephant - .... - ....

Egg - Goat - .... - ....

Turtle - Eagle - .... - ....

Lamp - Pencil - .... - ....

Lemon - Napkin - .... - ....

Keys

Outsider 1

Y	Y	Y	Y
Y	Y	Y	**T**
Y	Y	Y	Y
Y	Y	Y	Y

Outsider 2

Q	Q	Q	Q
Q	Q	Q	Q
Q	Q	Q	**O**
Q	Q	Q	Q

Outsider 3

b	b	b	b	b
b	b	b	b	b
b	b	b	**d**	b
b	b	b	b	b
b	b	b	b	b

Outsider 4

j	j	j	j	j
j	j	j	j	j
j	j	j	j	**i**
j	j	j	j	j
j	j	j	j	j

Keys

Outsider 5

w	w	w	w	w
w	w	w	w	w
w	w	w	w	w
w	w	w	w	w
w	w	v	w	w
w	w	w	w	w

Outsider 6

6	6	6	6	6	6	6
6	6	6	6	6	6	6
6	6	6	6	6	6	6
6	6	6	6	6	6	6
6	9	6	6	6	6	6
6	6	6	6	6	6	6
6	6	6	6	6	6	6
6	6	6	6	6	6	6

Before and After

a) 5-6-7

b) 2-3-4

c) 4-5-6

d) 11-12-13

e) 17-18-19

f) 6-7-8

g) 10-11-12

h) 2-3-4

i) 7-8-9

j) 3-4-5

k) 1-2-3

Lost Dots

a)

b)

c)

d)

e)

f)

g)

h)

i)

j)

Find the differences

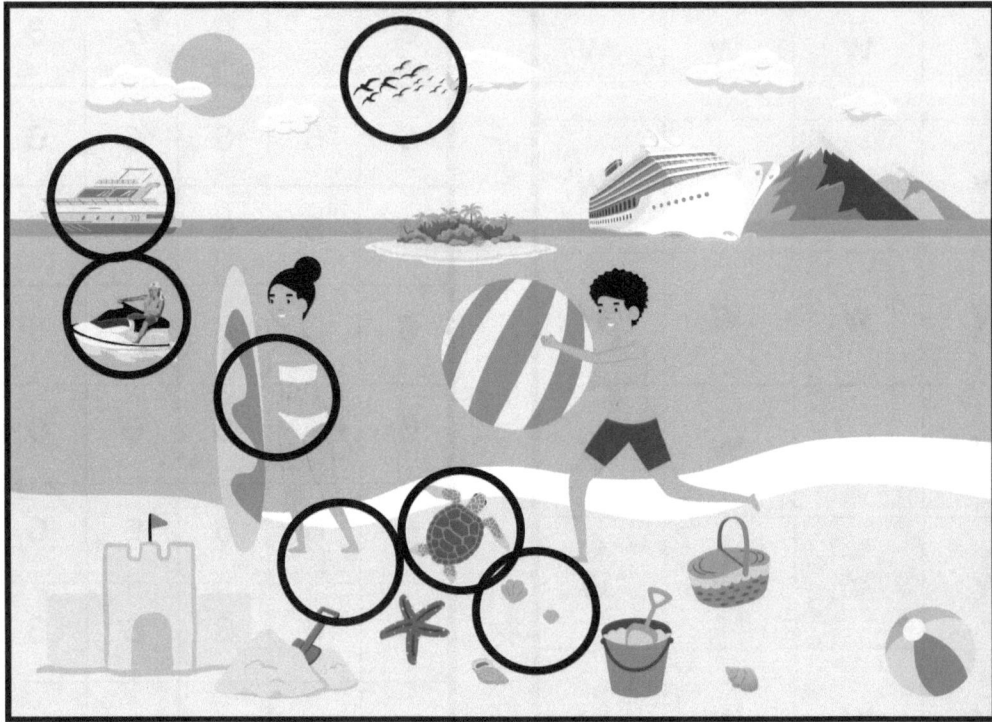

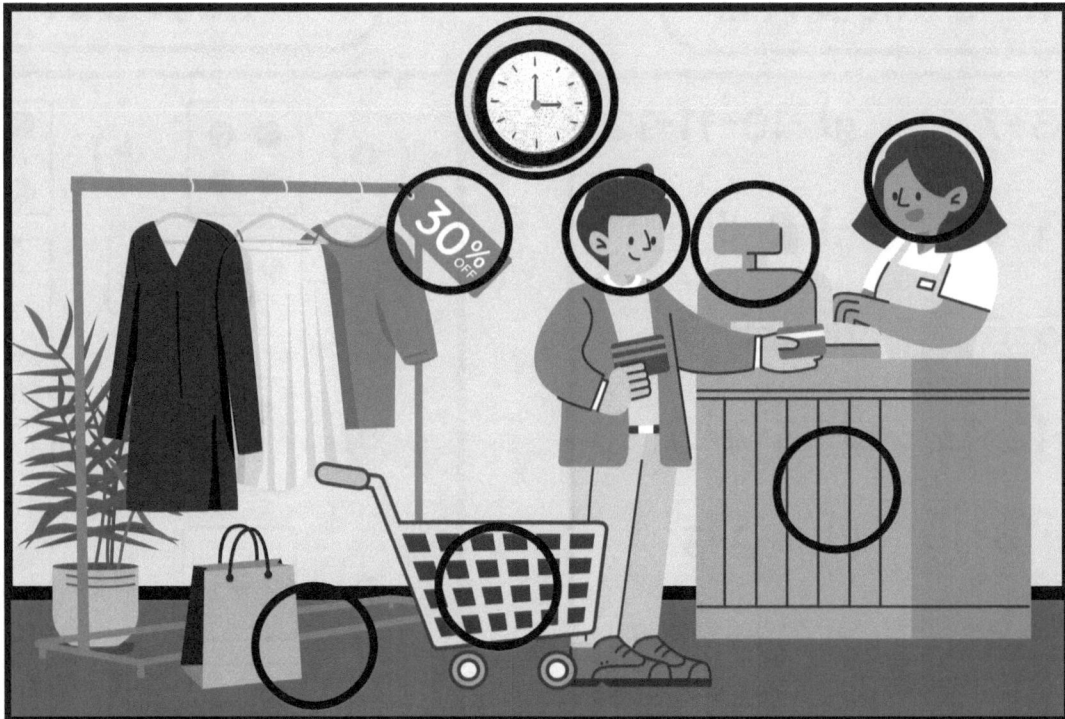

Keys

Word Search 1

D	P	C	T	F	D	B	E	F	K	X	N
V	Y	N	Z	K	R	F	S	T	W	B	V
S	T	N	W	A	L	K	T	R	L	A	D
R	S	P	U	B	N	W	A	E	V	L	O
C	U	G	W	P	P	U	N	A	H	A	X
N	E	K	Q	D	Q	Y	D	C	R	N	U
U	Z	Q	R	P	J	B	Q	H	Y	C	J
I	Y	C	D	Z	L	O	T	D	P	E	U
T	Z	G	E	O	W	H	A	H	L	N	D
S	T	R	E	T	C	H	G	V	G	N	P
P	X	I	C	H	H	L	L	U	P	O	W
S	V	P	H	B	E	H	D	L	B	W	Z

GRIP   WALK   STAND
REACH   BALANCE   STRETCH

Word Search 2

R	E	M	E	M	B	E	R	G	V	S	W	V
N	P	P	R	Q	Y	I	E	Y	X	Y	F	O
Q	A	V	C	M	P	C	C	B	X	B	X	G
D	R	K	D	S	P	E	A	K	J	Q	B	L
G	V	A	S	C	M	E	L	G	Z	B	B	I
N	Y	T	I	H	Z	P	L	V	W	E	O	S
A	Y	K	R	B	R	Z	Y	L	F	E	L	T
L	K	U	V	J	E	A	U	M	L	V	D	E
Q	M	K	T	A	A	C	Y	T	P	B	C	N
S	M	F	K	U	D	E	J	I	I	R	P	Y
U	A	W	X	G	W	R	I	T	E	G	H	H
T	K	W	U	H	E	N	X	P	K	S	M	A
V	A	X	Z	M	P	Y	X	T	Q	P	Q	U

READ   SPEAK   WRITE
LISTEN   RECALL   REMEMBER

Word Search 3

U	A	B	R	E	A	T	H	E	W	F	N
B	Z	K	E	S	C	R	U	W	M	K	P
P	F	S	L	E	E	P	V	X	J	X	Q
L	E	Z	A	D	K	R	L	M	U	F	B
G	D	S	X	O	F	D	G	T	Z	G	P
P	C	B	L	N	O	S	R	M	T	X	X
X	A	P	X	O	D	V	E	Z	O	Y	D
K	L	U	R	A	F	X	S	D	D	Y	O
H	M	X	U	S	E	D	T	Y	A	J	R
S	L	N	F	A	E	K	A	L	I	N	U
J	O	S	T	I	L	C	B	K	D	K	F
I	G	N	Y	S	X	A	Y	N	G	A	I

FEEL   REST   CALM
RELAX   SLEEP   BREATHE

Word Search 4

I	W	X	H	G	A	N	X	Z	Q	H	O	I
P	J	A	F	I	V	F	N	W	H	M	R	X
L	E	A	R	N	T	P	S	N	M	Q	T	S
A	W	B	C	Q	W	R	I	L	E	Z	H	M
N	X	I	K	S	H	A	O	Z	T	T	I	J
J	H	V	B	O	G	C	T	V	T	J	N	Q
R	W	R	H	L	F	T	D	D	Q	H	K	N
A	H	Q	N	V	H	I	W	C	J	W	D	R
Z	X	C	G	E	C	C	I	Z	L	A	N	O
V	J	O	T	G	D	E	U	A	G	A	S	Z
X	E	C	C	Q	S	C	H	O	O	S	E	N
S	D	F	M	E	T	U	P	Q	F	G	L	K
H	N	G	E	M	C	O	E	M	R	V	Z	O

PLAN   THINK   SOLVE
LEARN   CHOOSE   PRACTICE

Keys

Egg Sequence
c), a) and b)

Sunflower Sequence
c), b), a) and d)

Routine 1: Getting Ready for Bed
1. Change into pajamas.
2. Use the bathroom to brush your teeth and wash your face.
3. Turn off lights and other electronics in the house.
4. Get into bed and set the alarm for the morning.

Routine 2: Preparing to Go to the Grocery Store
1. Write a shopping list of needed items.
2. Put on a coat and shoes.
3. Grab reusable shopping bags and the list.
4. Lock the door behind you as you leave the house.

Routine 3: Making a Cup of Tea
1. Fill the kettle with water and turn it on.
2. Choose a teabag and place it in the cup.
3. Pour the hot water into the cup once the kettle is boiling.
4. Let the tea steep for a few minutes before drinking.

Keys

Routine 4: Watching a Favorite TV Show

1. Turn on the television and select the correct channel.
2. Sit down on a comfortable chair or sofa.
3. Use the remote to set the volume to a comfortable level.
4. Find the show in the TV guide and watch it at the scheduled time.

Matching 1

Musical Instruments – Guitar
Furniture – Chair
Vehicles – Bicycle
Professions – Doctor
Tools – Hammer
Foods – Pasta

Matching 2

Flowers – Rose
Sports – Tennis
Fruits – Apple
Appliances – TV
Clothing – Shirt
Animals – Cat

Matching 3

BEACH
SCHOOL
KITCHEN
WEATHER
BODY PARTS

FRUITS

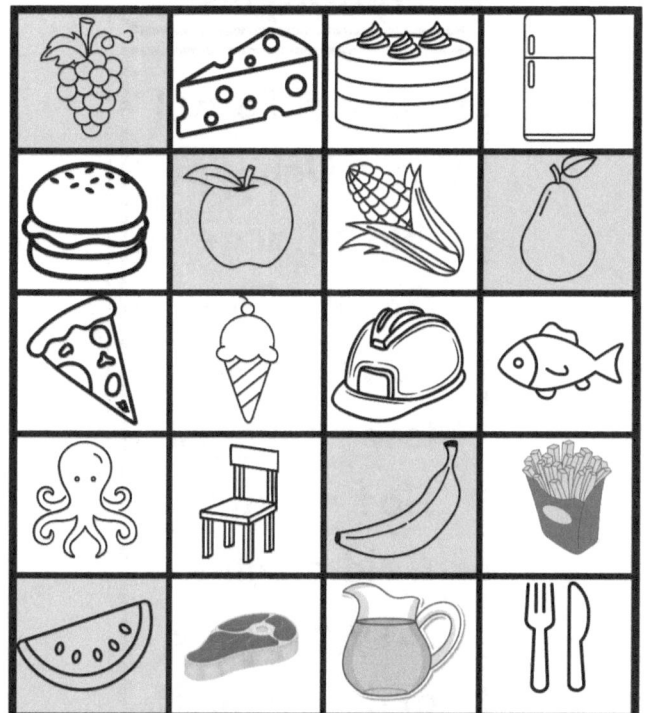

45

Keys

ANIMALS

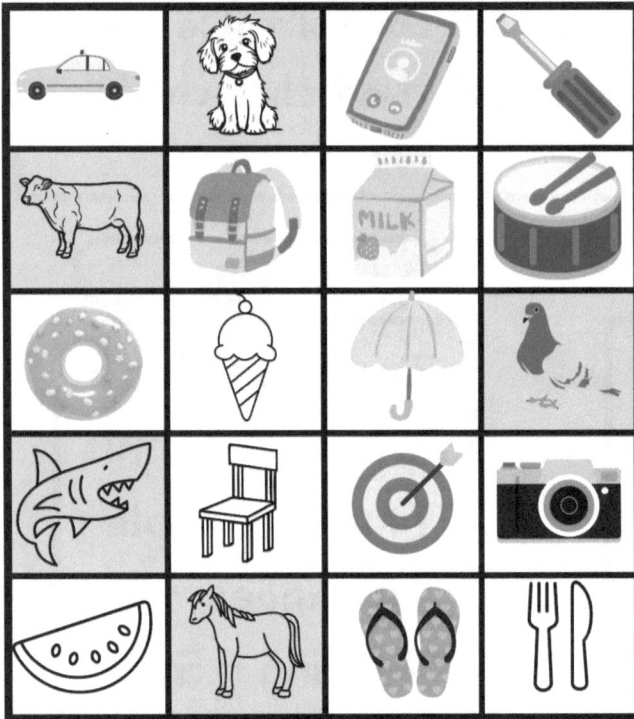

FAMILY

CARD	GRANDSON	OVEN	DOCTOR
HEATING	COFFEE	DAUGHTER	PIZZA
DOOR	MOTHER	CUP	GARDEN
UNCLE	PHONE	PEN	FLOOR
TAXI	HOSPITAL	WIFE	BOTTLE

Synonyms

Happy – Joyful
Sad – Unhappy
Big – Large
Small – Tiny
Fast – Quick
Slow – Sluggish
Hot – Warm
Cold – Chilly
Easy – Simple
Hard – Difficult

Antonyms

Old – New
Tall – Short
Rich – Poor
Smart – Dumb
Full – Empty
Good – Bad
Pretty – Ugly
Wet – Dry
Near – Far
High – Low

Keys

Word Associaton 1

SUN – LIGHT
MOON – NIGHT
STARS – SKY
OCEAN – WAVES
BEACH – SAND
FLOWER – GARDEN
TREE – LEAVES
SLEEP – BED

Word Associaton 2

COFFEE – MORNING
TEA – AFTERNOON
MEAL – RESTAURANT
GLASSES – VISION
COMPUTER – TECHNOLOGY
PHONE – CALL
LETTER – MAIL
KEY – LOCK

Connection 1

0 – ZERO
3 – THREE
5 – FIVE
8 – EIGHT
12 – TWELVE
17 – SEVENTEEN
19 – NINETEEN
23 – TWENTY-THREE

Connection 2

1 – ONE
4 – FOUR
6 – SIX
9 – NINE
13 – THIRTEEN
15 – FIFTEEN
18 – EIGHTEEN
22 – TWENTY-TWO

Spatial and Visual Skills

-Mazes and Puzzles

-Pattern Tracking

-Visual Tracking

★ **Usefulness:**

Improved Visual Perception
Enhanced Spatial Awareness
Stronger Hand-Eye Coordination
Boosted Independent Living Skills

INSTRUCTIONS

📌 It is advised not to use a highlighter as it could bleed through the page.

📌 In some statements, the explanation of the exercise is highlighted. In these cases, it involves an additional task to be performed to increase the difficulty of the exercise.

📌 The solutions are found at the end of each section.

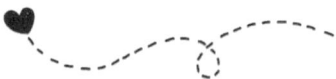

Shadow Matching

Connect each object with its corresponding shadow.

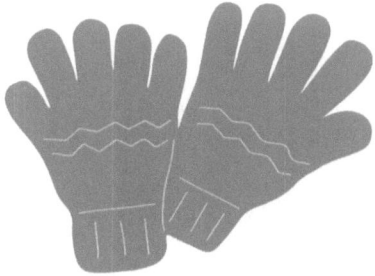

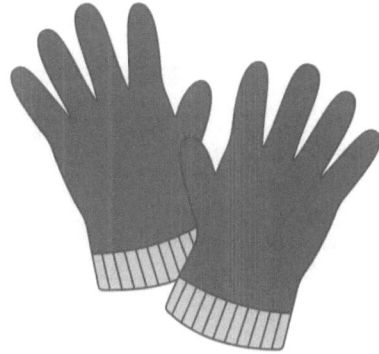

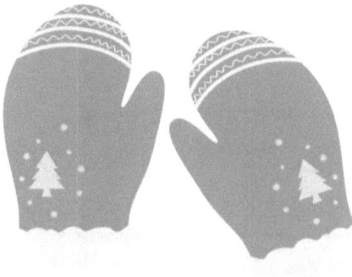

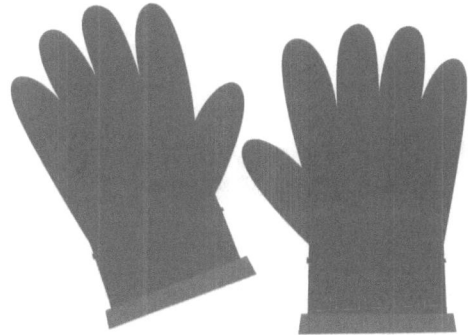

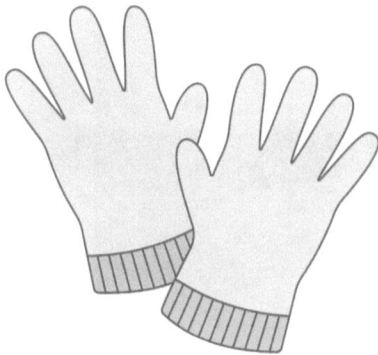

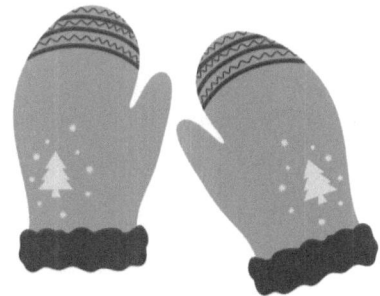

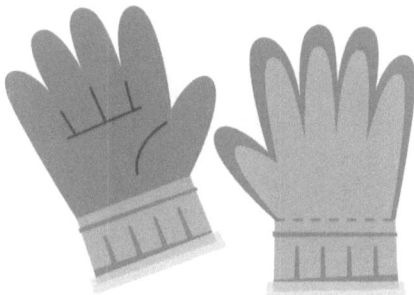

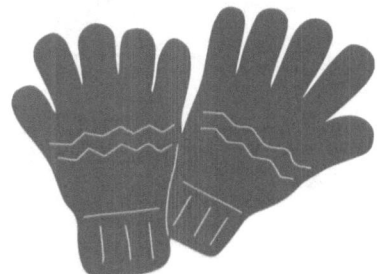

Shadow Matching

Connect each object with its corresponding shadow.

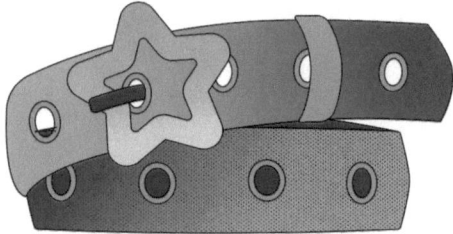

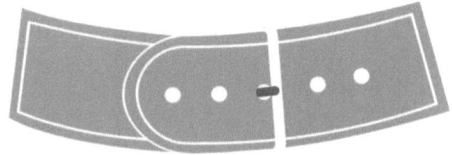

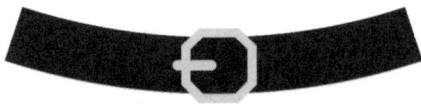

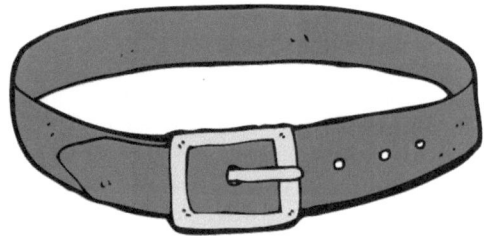

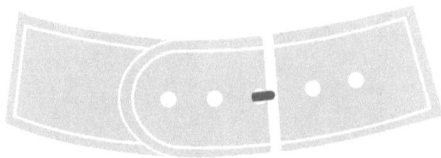

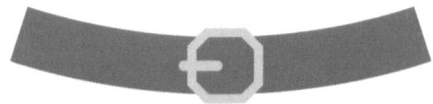

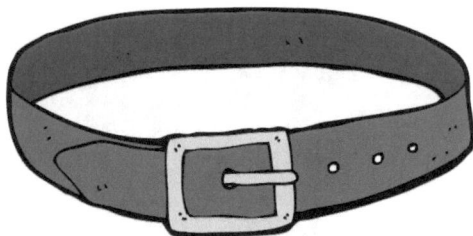

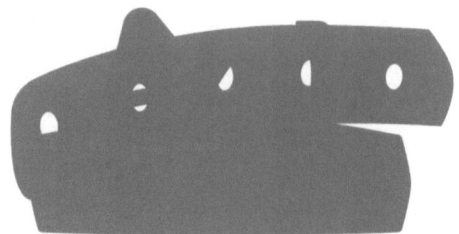

Shadow Matching

Connect each object with its corresponding shadow.

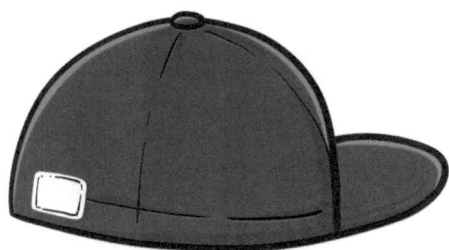

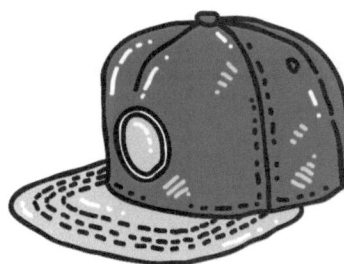

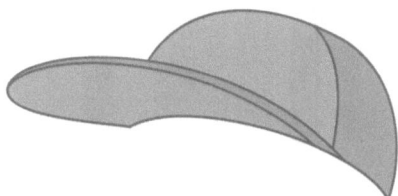

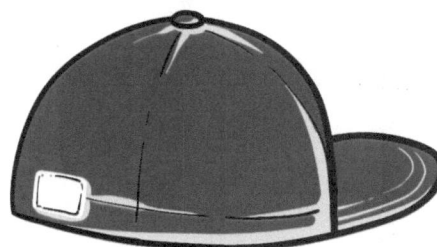

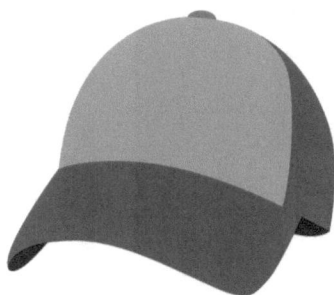

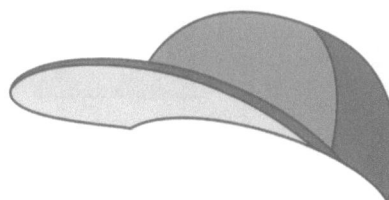

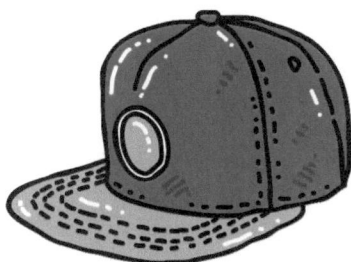

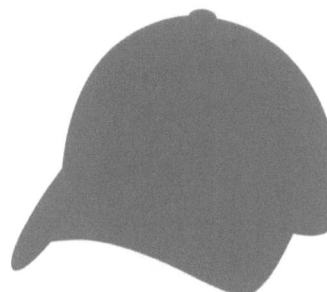

Maze

Help Olivia to find Liam.

Maze

Help the doctor to find the hospital.

Maze

Help the miner to find gold.

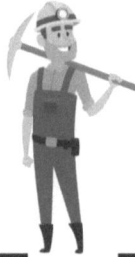

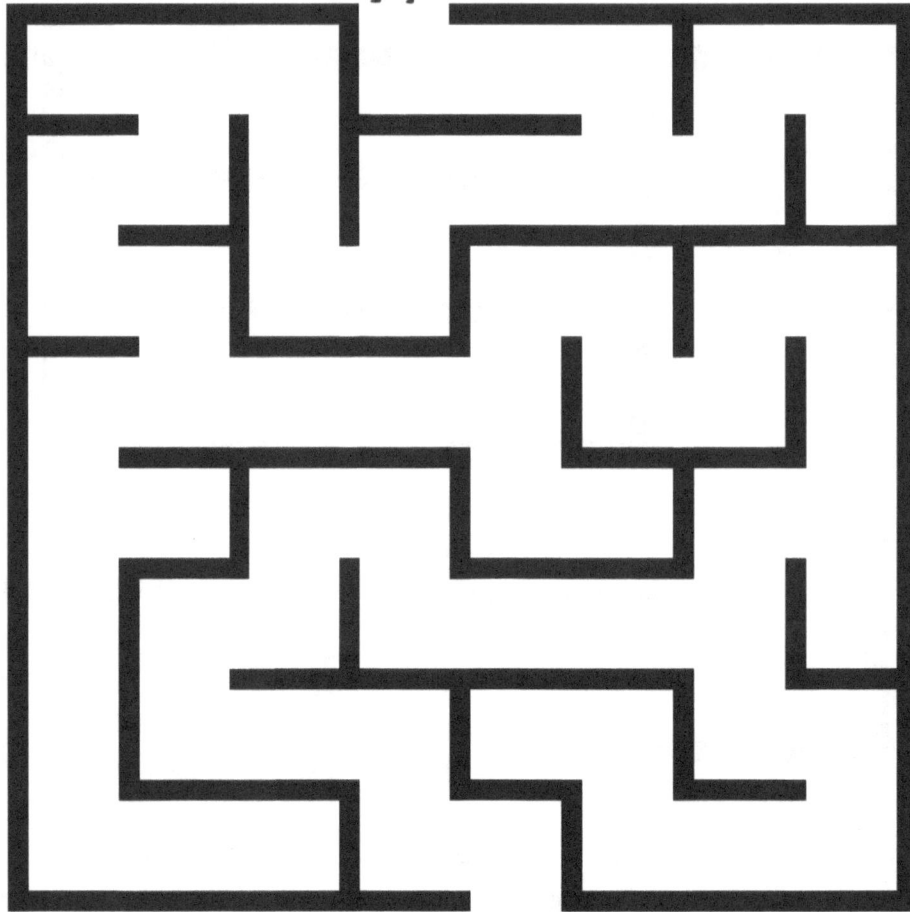

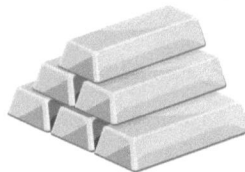

Maze

Help Marcus to find the bank.

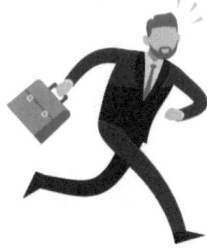

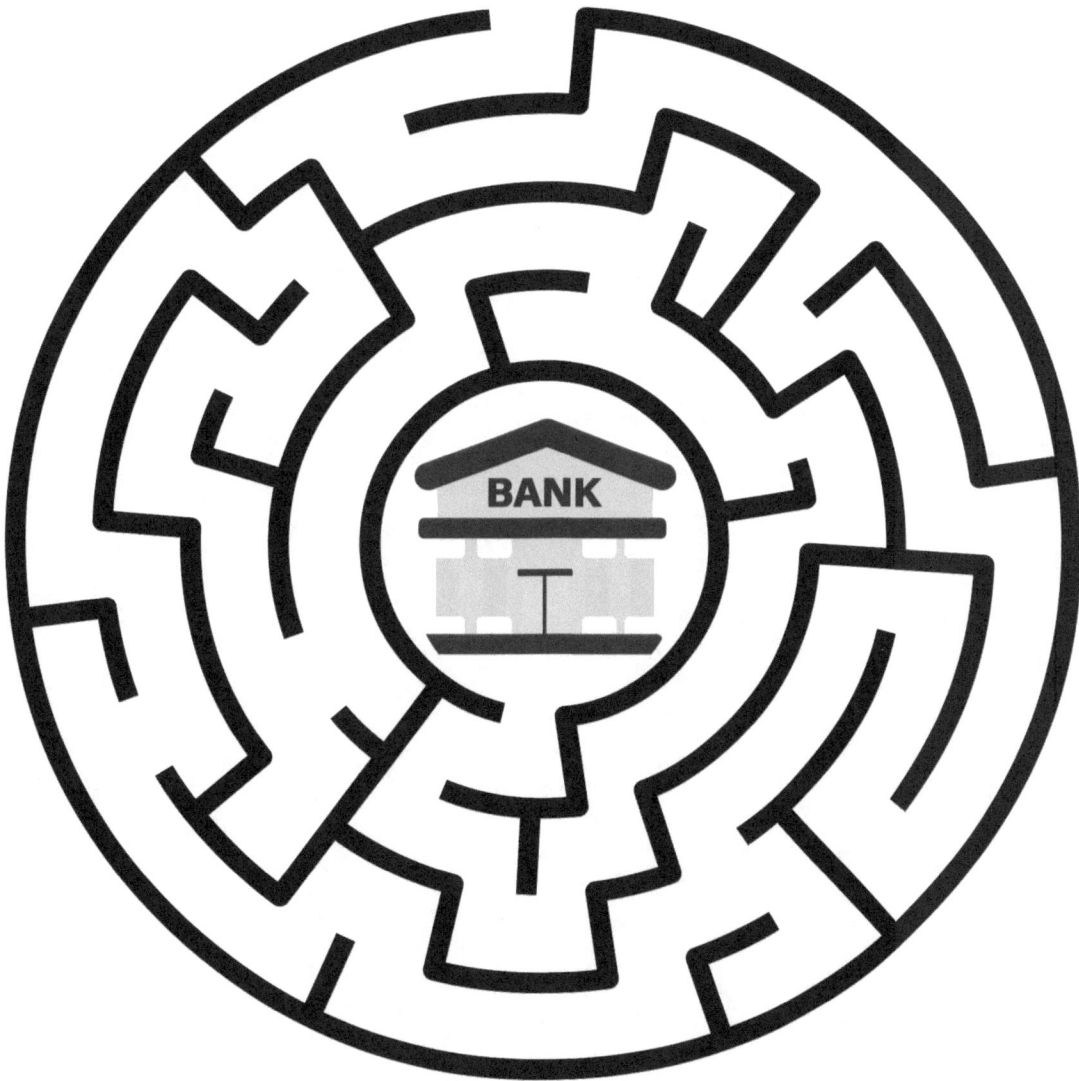

Maze

Help James to
find the park.

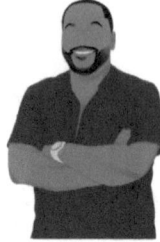

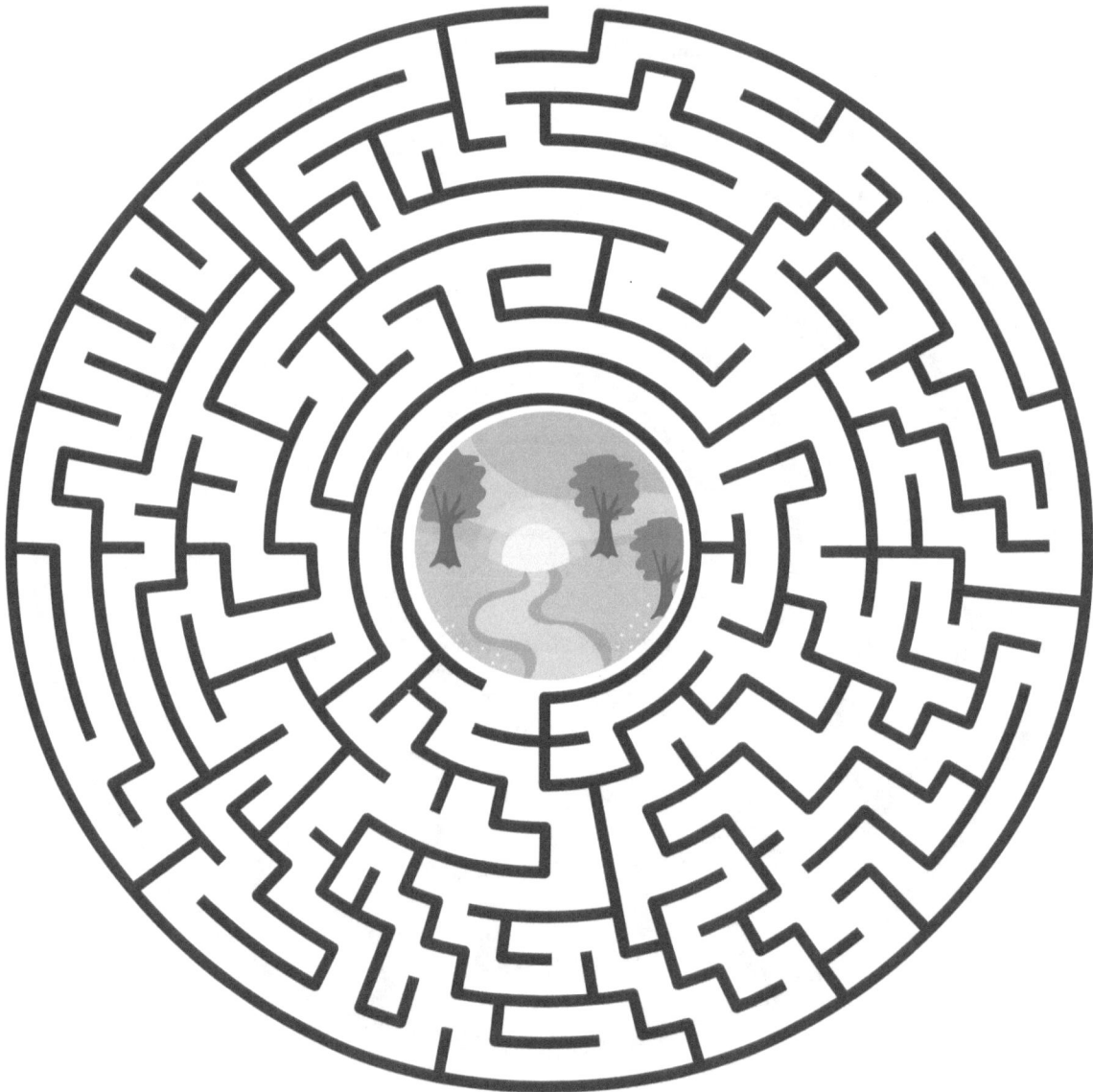

What comes next?

Observe the patterned block and choose which option comes next.

a)
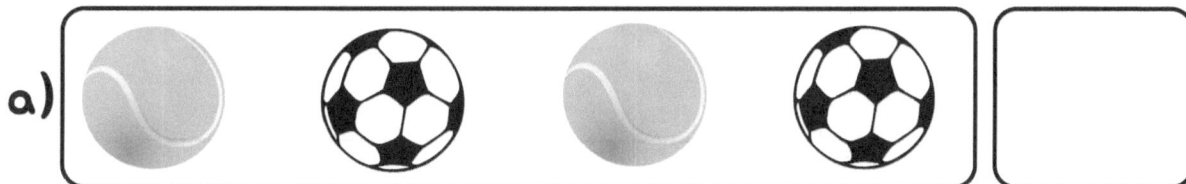

b)

c)
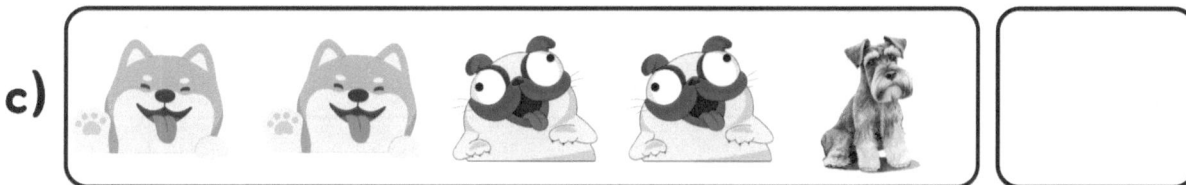

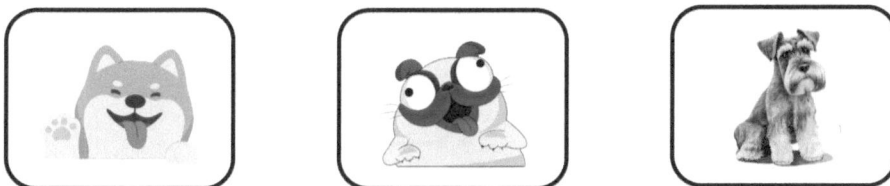

What comes next?

Observe the patterned block and choose which option comes next.

d) [sponge] [shower] [shower] [sponge] [shower] [ ]

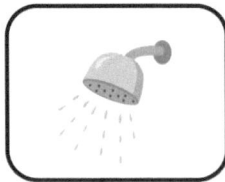 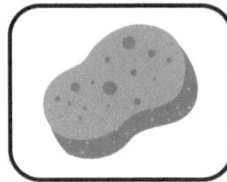

e) [grandma] [girl] [woman] [grandma] [ ]

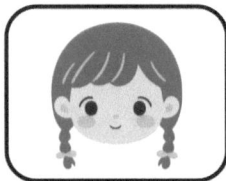 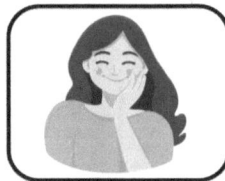 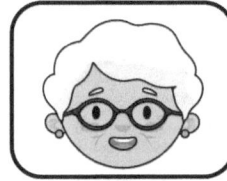

f) [tooth] [toothbrush] [tooth] [toothbrush] [ ]

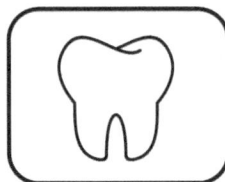 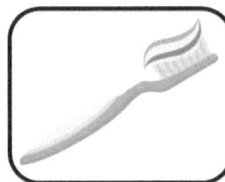

What comes next?

Observe the patterned block and choose which option comes next.

g)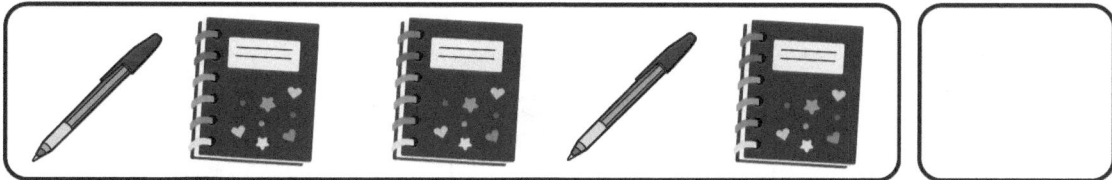

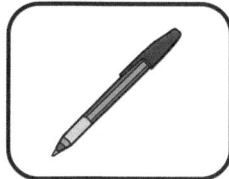 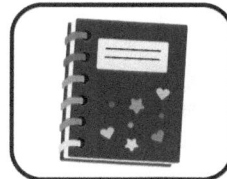

h)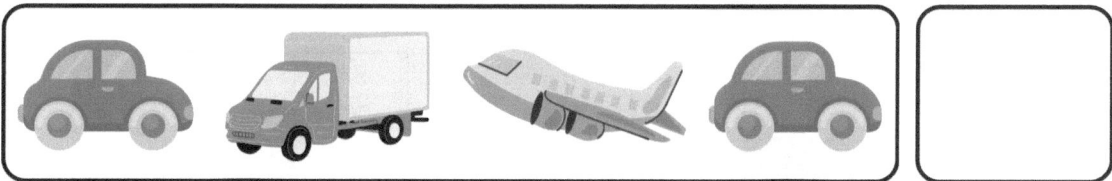

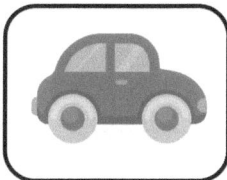 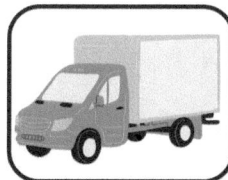 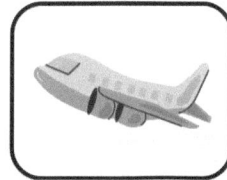

i)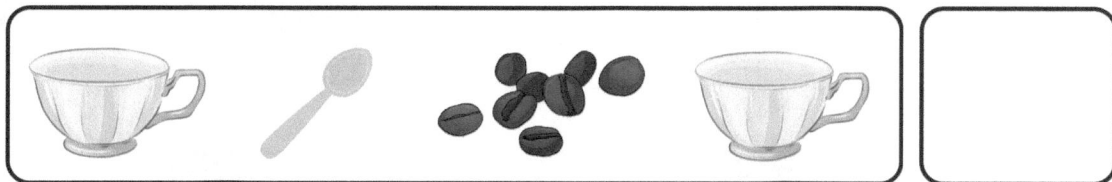

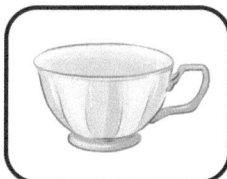 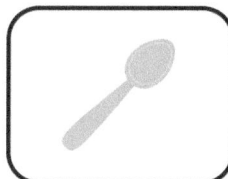 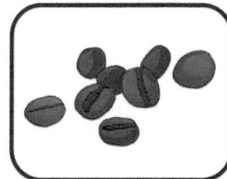

Which is the next?

Observe the patterned block and choose which option comes next.

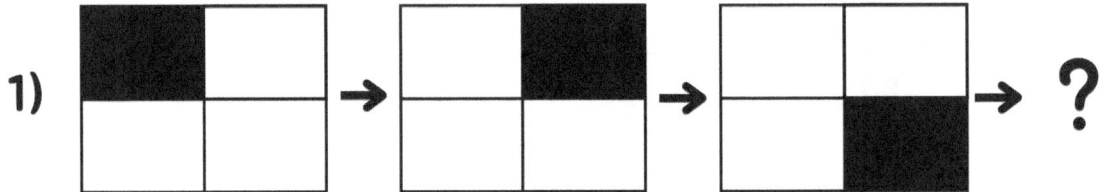

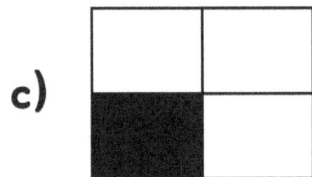

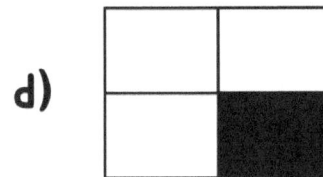

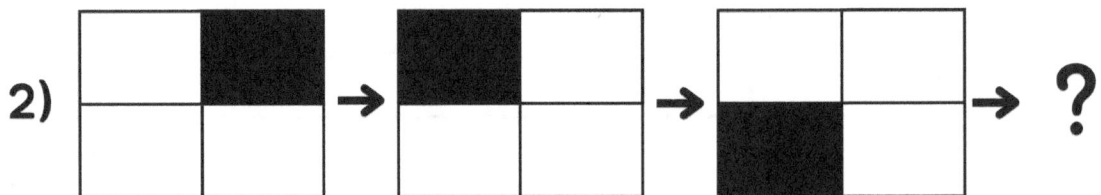

1) → → → **?**

a)

b)

c)

d)

2) → → → **?**

a)

b)

c)

d)

Which is the next?

Observe the patterned block and choose which option comes next.

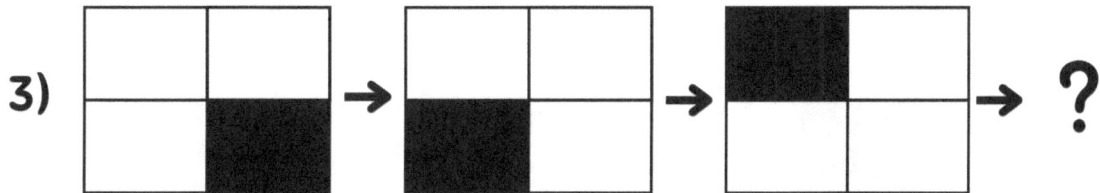

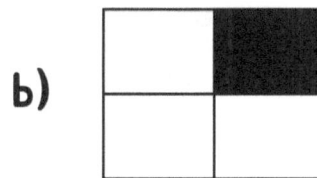

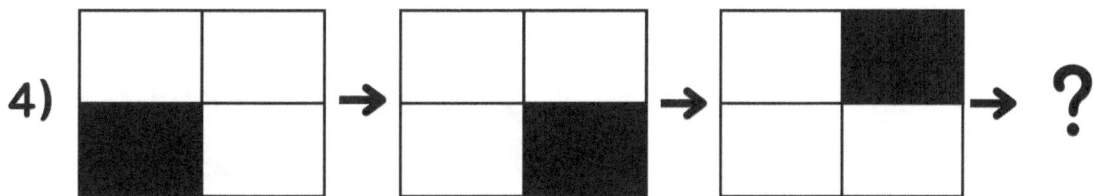

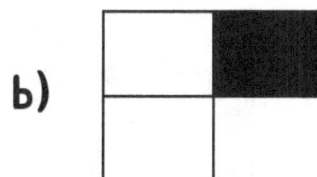

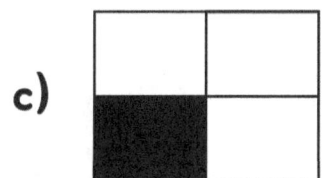

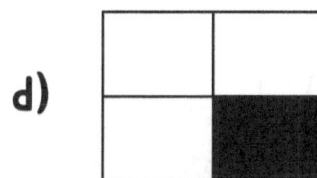

3)

a)

b)

c)

d)

4)

a)

b)

c)

d)

Which is the next?

Observe the patterned block and choose which option comes next.

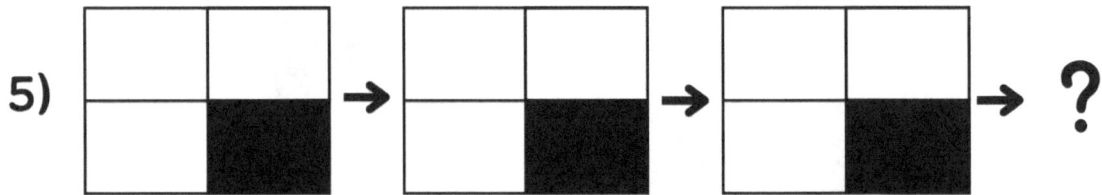

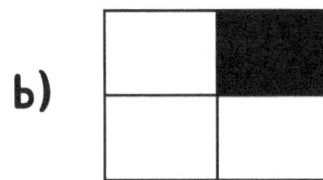

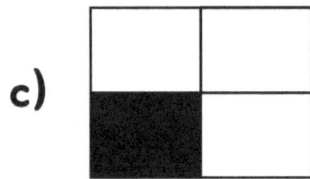

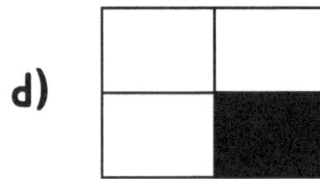

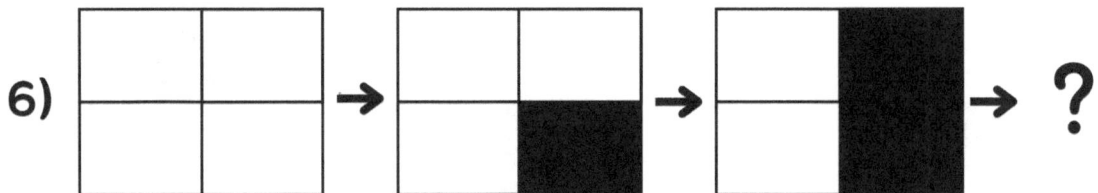

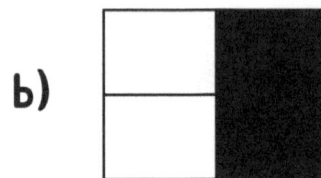

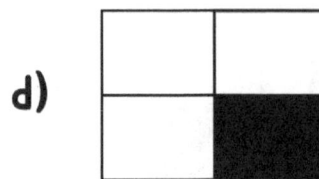

5) → → → ?

a)

b)

c)

d)

6) → → → ?

a)

b)

c)

d)

Which is the next?

Observe the patterned block and choose which option comes next.

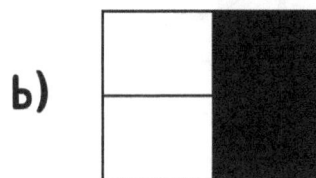

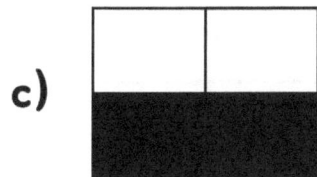

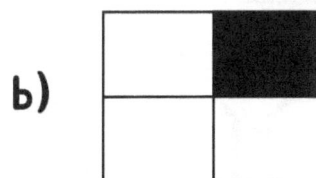

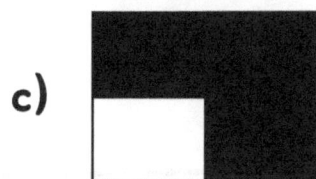

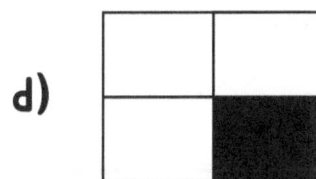

7) → → → ?

a)

b)

c)

d)

8) → → → ?

a)

b)

c)

d)

Finish the Pattern

Observe the patterned block and draw which option comes next.
You can also color them.

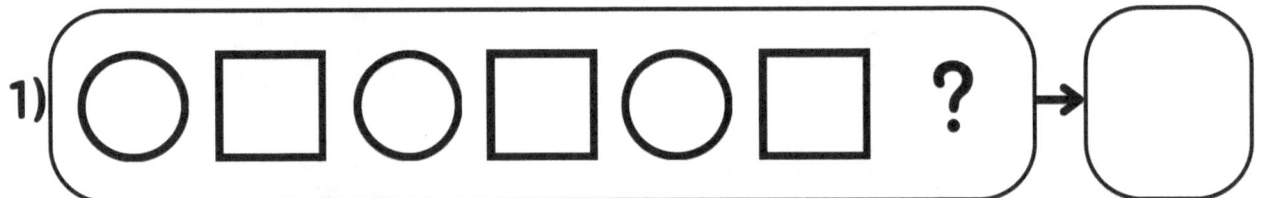

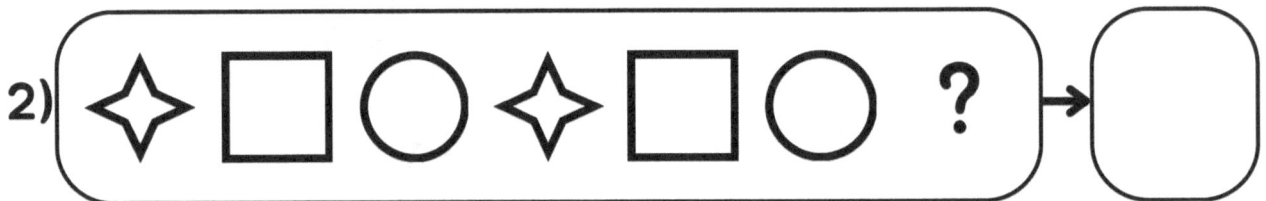

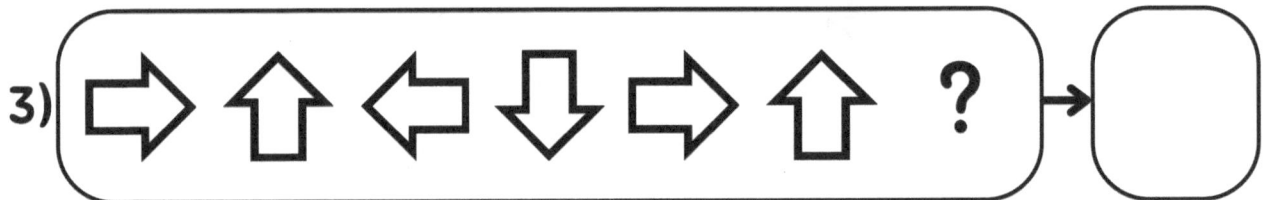

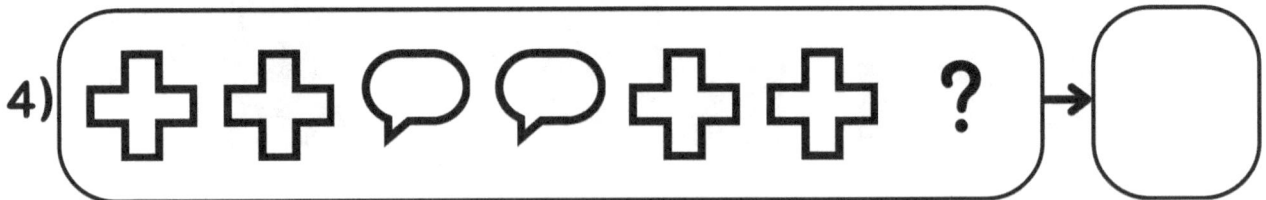

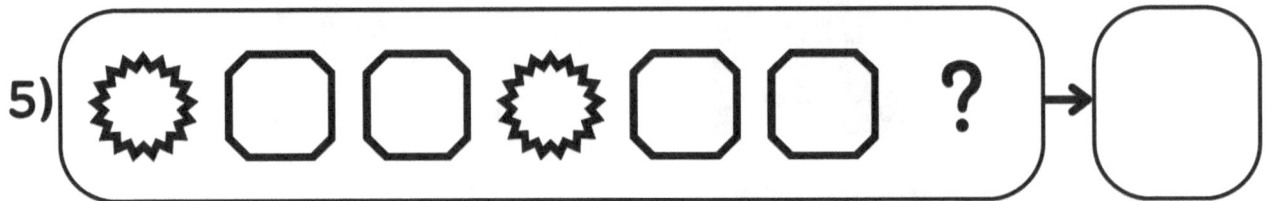

1) ○ □ ○ □ ○ □ ? →

2) ✦ □ ○ ✦ □ ○ ? →

3) ➡ ⬆ ⬅ ⬇ ➡ ⬆ ? →

4) ✚ ✚ 💬 💬 ✚ ✚ ? →

5) ✺ ⬡ ⬡ ✺ ⬡ ⬡ ? →

Finish the Pattern

Observe the patterned block and draw which
option comes next.
You can also color them.

6) ⇒ ⇐ ⇔ ⇒ ⇐ ⇔ ? →

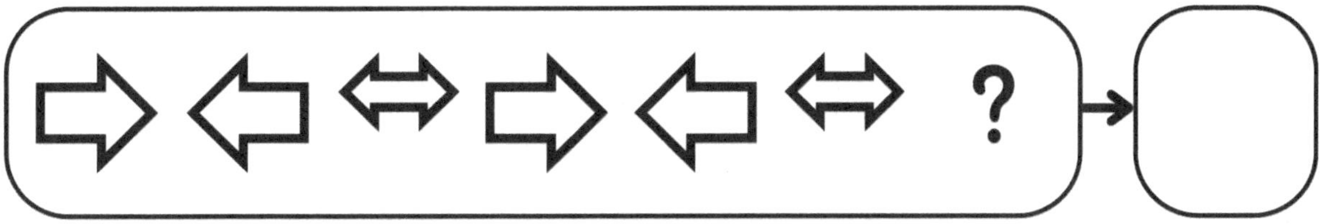

7) △ ▽ ◇ ◇ △ ▽ ? →

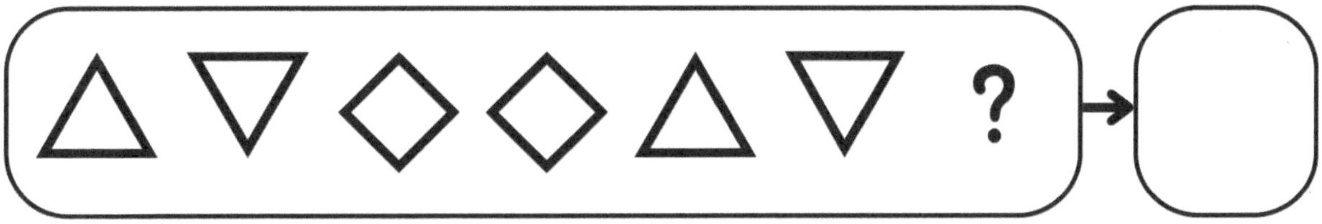

8) ✦ ☆ ✡ ✴ ✦ ☆ ? →

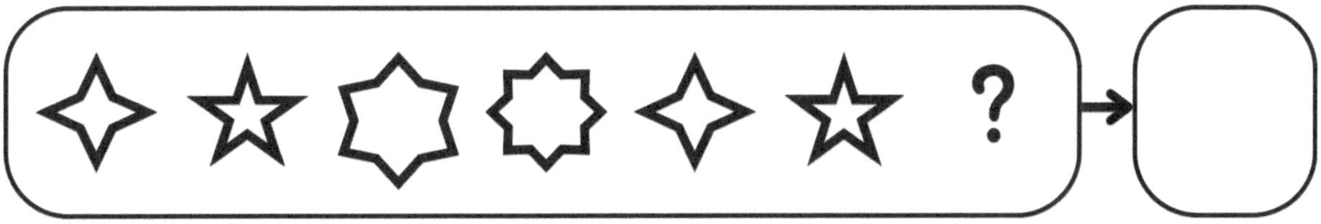

9) 💬 💬 ♡ 💬 💬 ♡ ? →

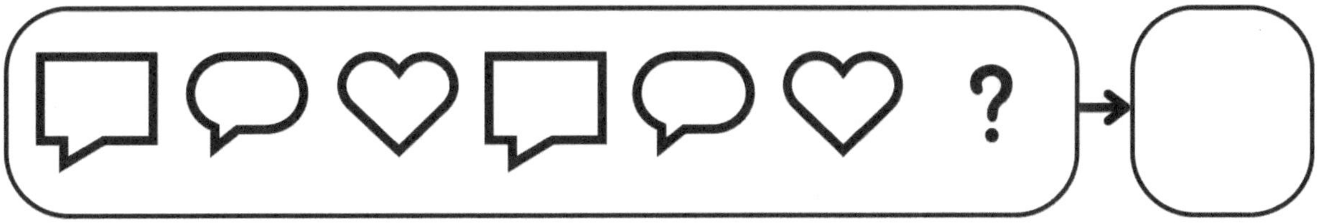

10) ◇ ◇ ◇ ⬡ ◇ ◇ ? →

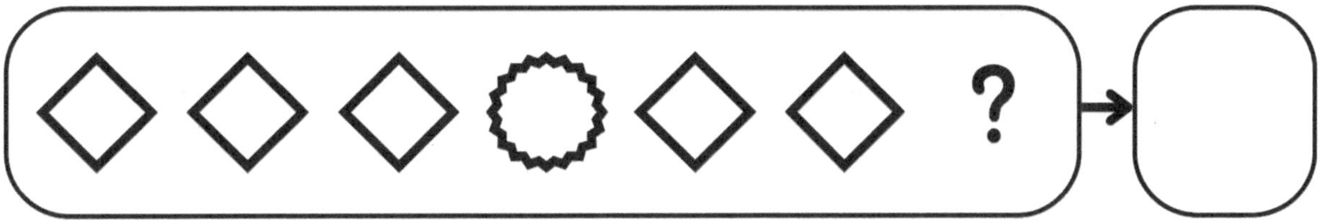

Which letter follows?

Observe the following letters and write the next one in the circle. Use the alphabet if necessary.

1)

D E F ( )

2)

S T U ( )

3)

A B C ( )

4)

O P Q ( )

5)

L M N ( )

6)

P Q R ( )

7)

H I J ( )

8)

V W X ( )

A B C D E F G H I J K L M
N O P Q R S T U V W X Y Z

Which letter follows?

Observe the following letters and write the next one in the circle. Use the alphabet if necessary.

9)

A   C   E   ( )

10)

H   J   L   ( )

11)

P   Q   S   ( )

12)

F   H   J   ( )

13)

C   F   I   ( )

14)

Z   Y   X   ( )

15)

K   M   O   ( )

16)

M   K   I   ( )

A B C D E F G H I J K L M
N O P Q R S T U V W X Y Z

Family Maze

Help grandparents find their grandchildren.

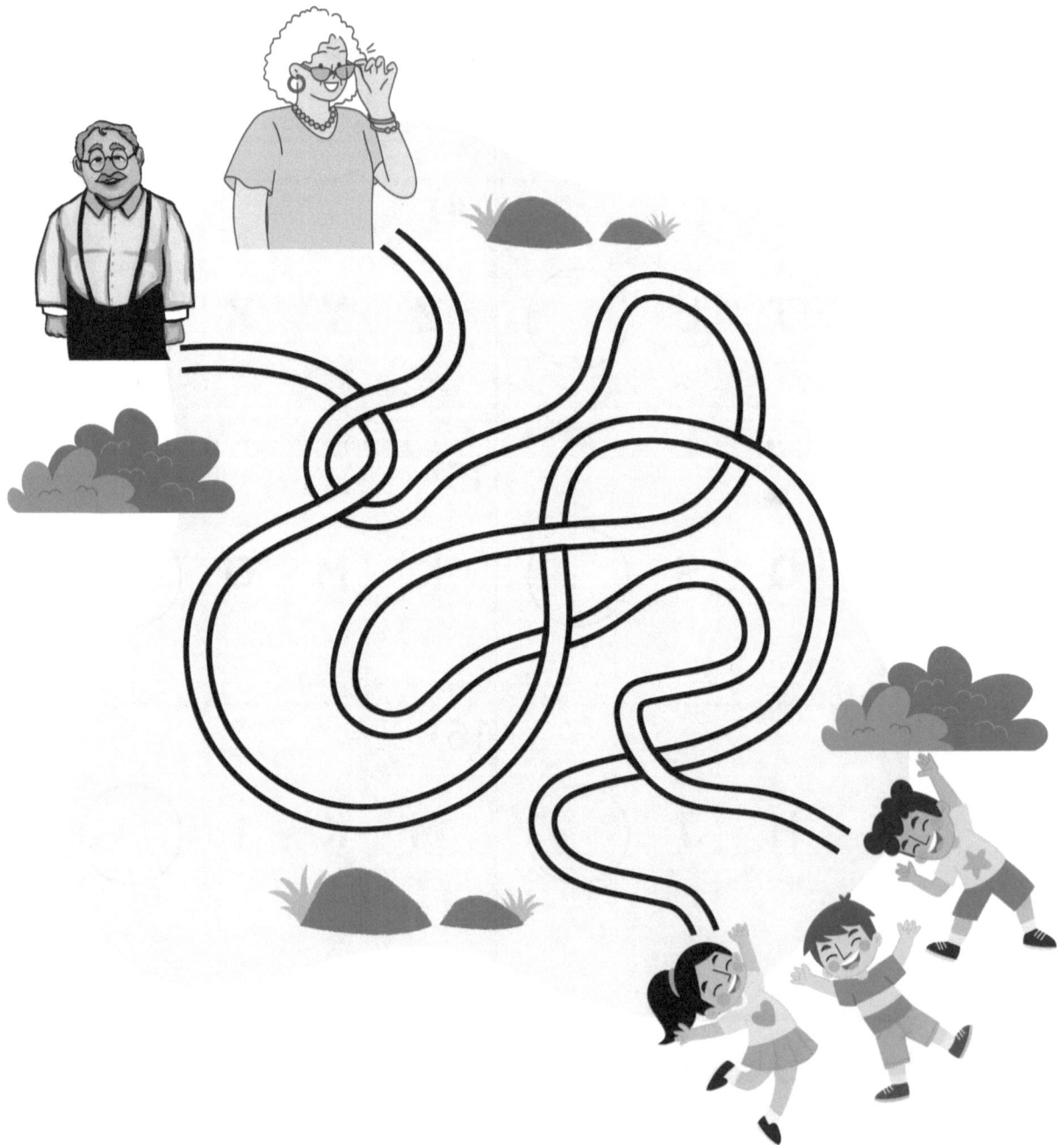

Emergency Workers Maze

Help the emergency worker find their vehicle.

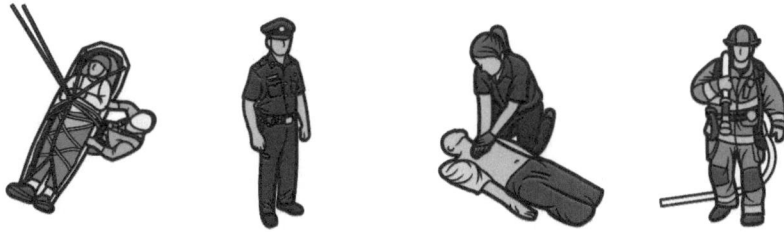

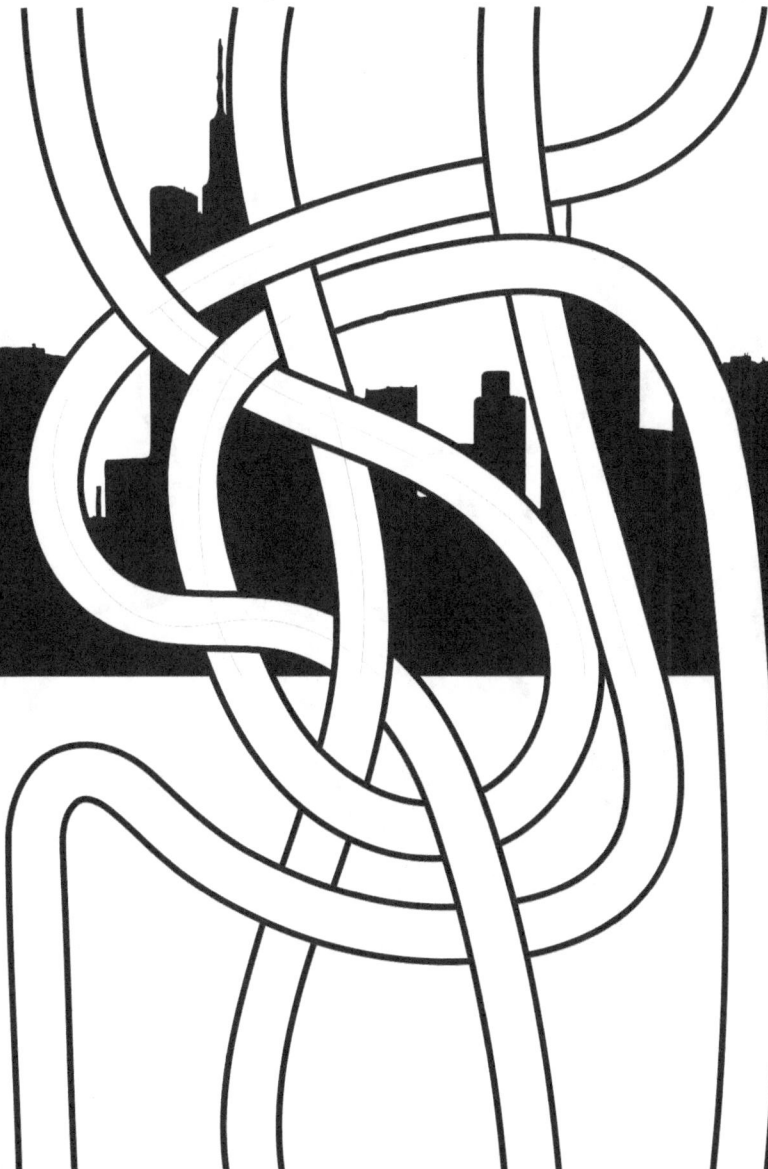

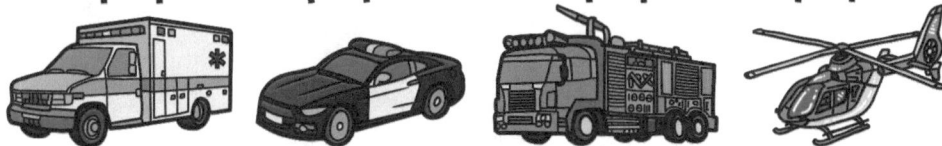

Jobs Maze

Help workers get to their jobs.

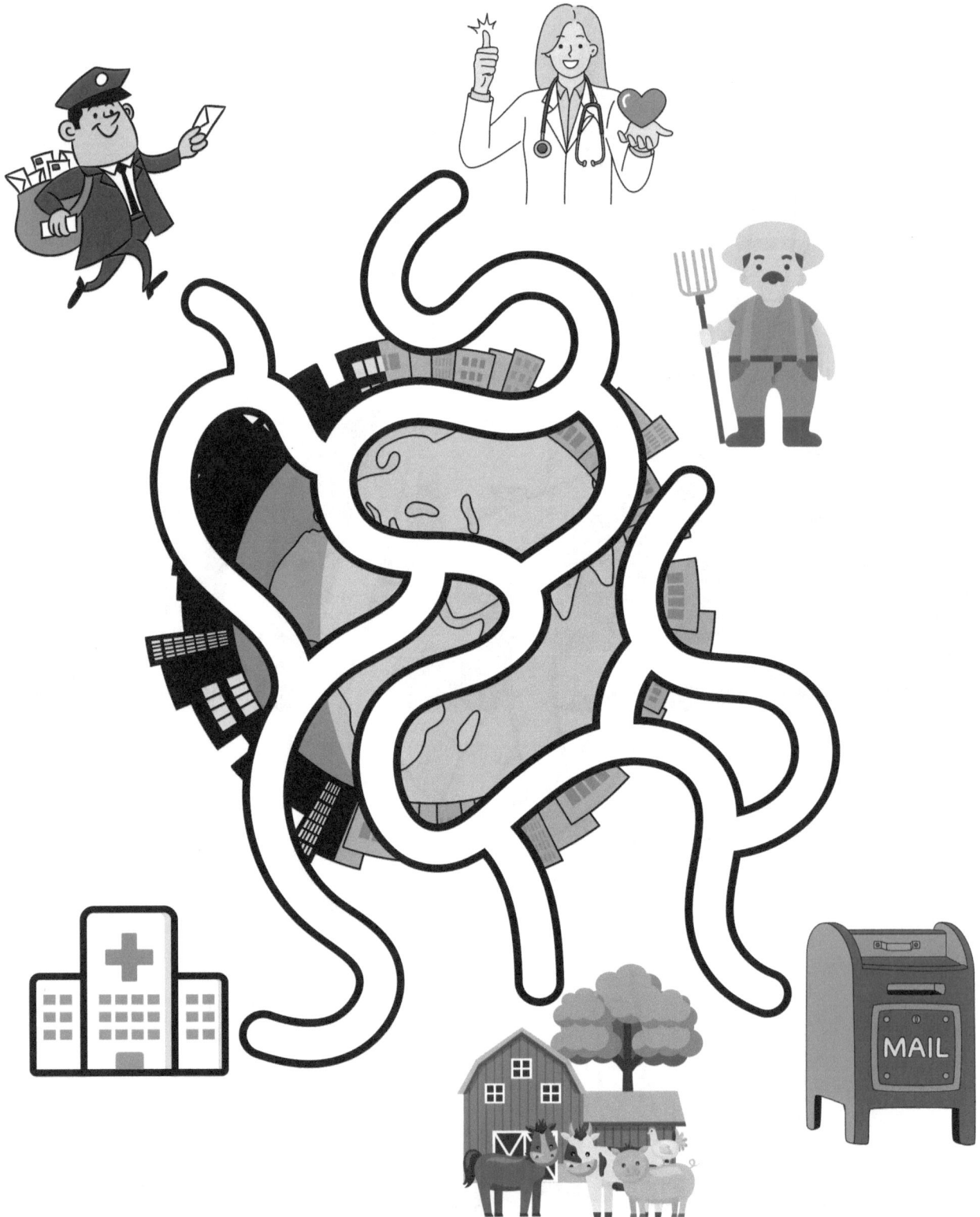

Recovery Maze

Help Linda go to therapy.

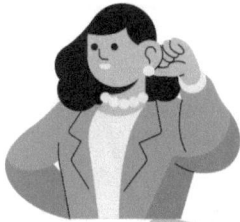

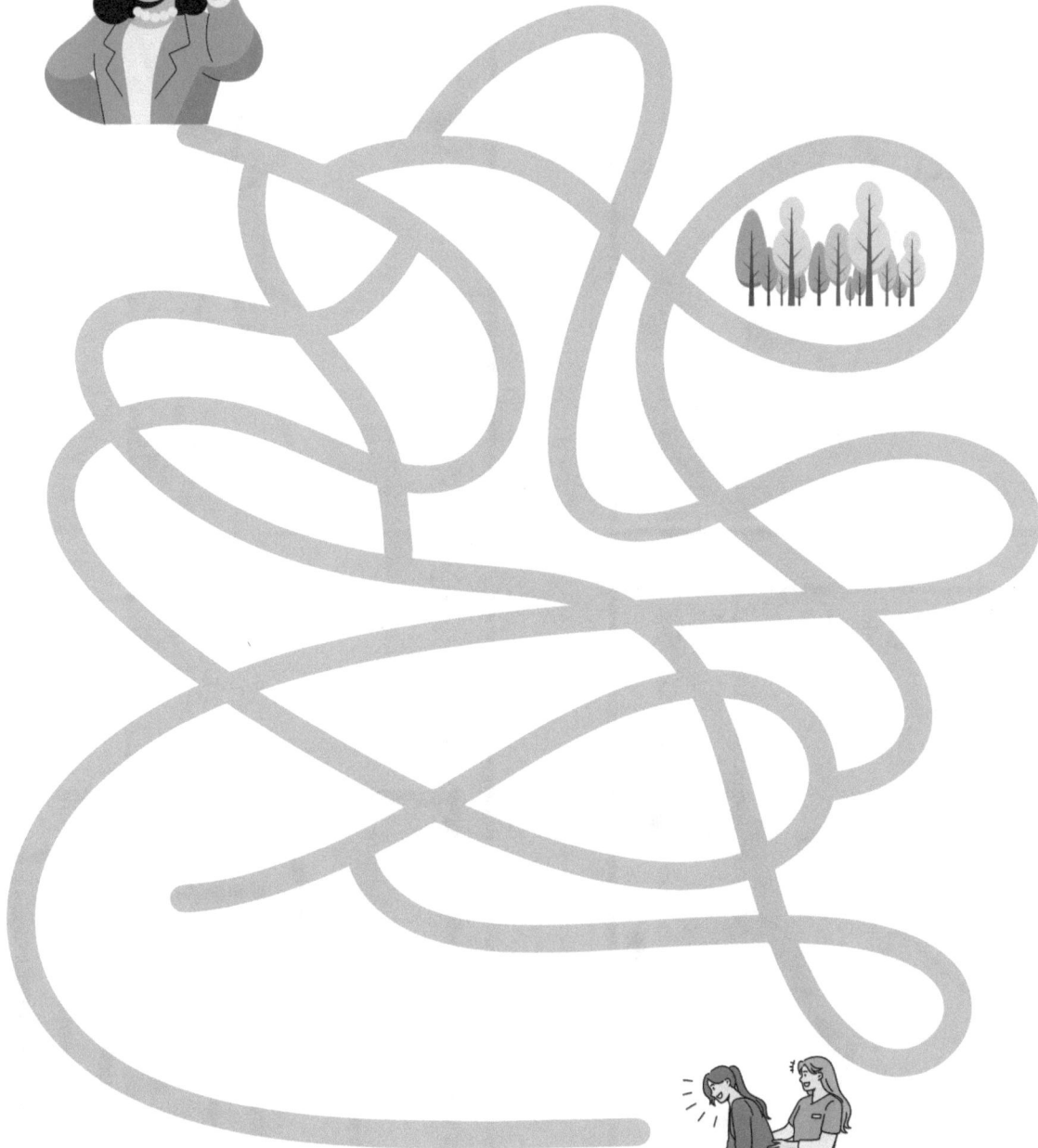

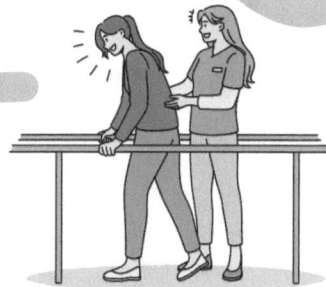

TOGETHER
* in *
RECOVERY

Keys

Shadow Matching Key

Shadow Matching Key

Shadow Matching Key

Maze Key

Keys

Maze Key

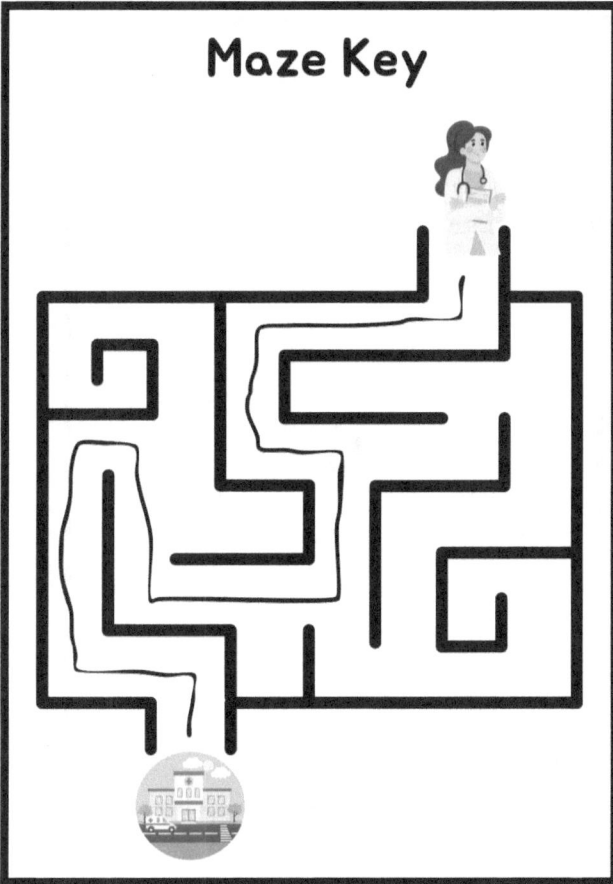

Maze Key

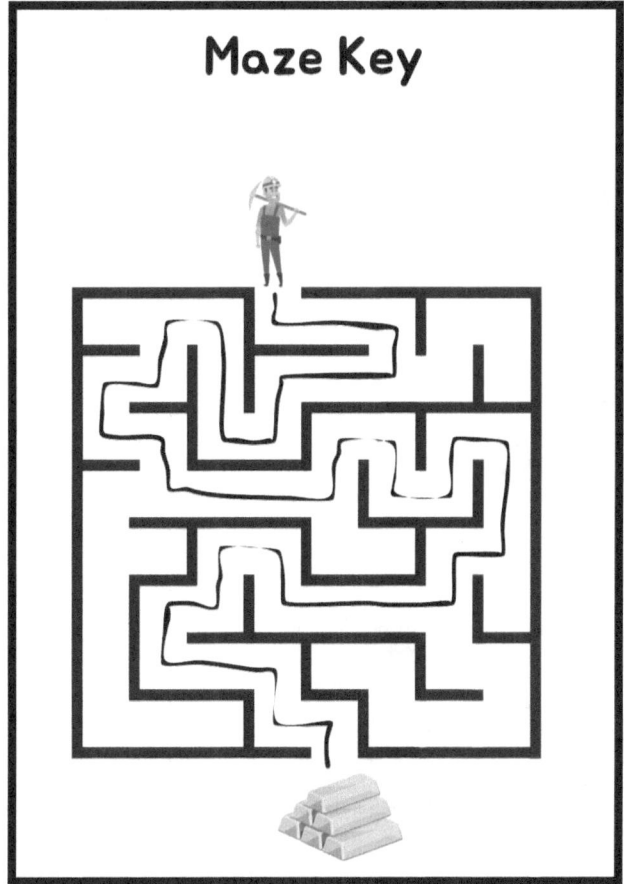

Maze Key

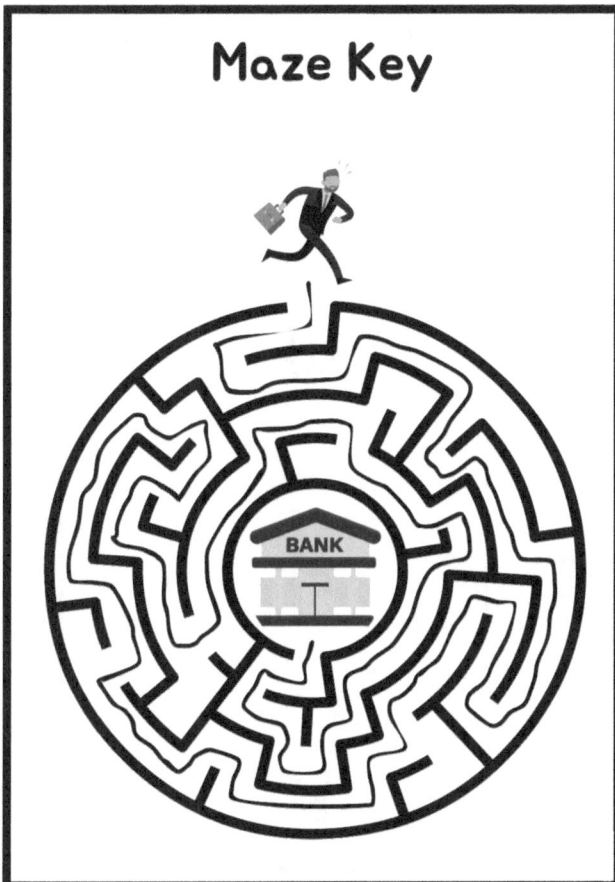

Maze Key

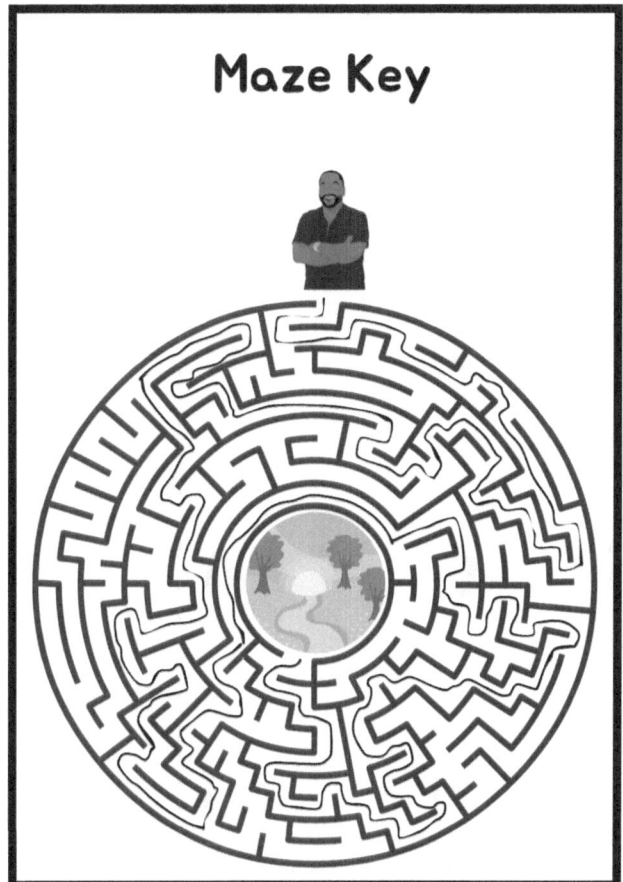

Keys

a)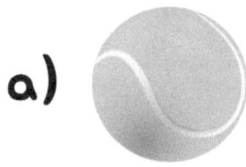

b)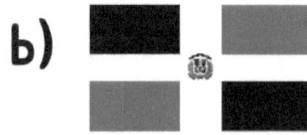

c)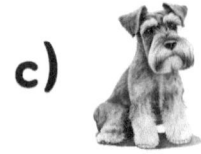

d)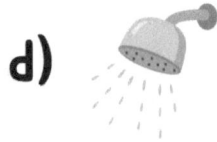

e)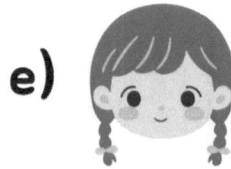

f)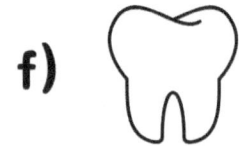

g)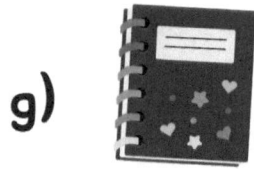

h)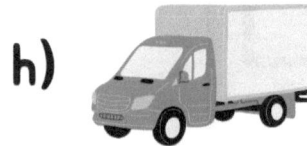

i)

Which is the next? Key

1)	c)	2)	d)
3)	b)	4)	a)
5)	d)	6)	c)
7)	a)	8)	b)

Keys

Finish the Pattern - Key

1) ⬭

2) ✦

3) ⬅

4) 💬

5) ✳

6) ➡

7) ◇

8) ✷

9) 🗩

10) ◇

Which letter follows? Key

1) G	5) O	9) G	13) L
2) V	7) S	10) N	14) W
3) D	7) K	11) V	15) Q
4) R	8) Y	12) L	16) G

Keys

Family Maze

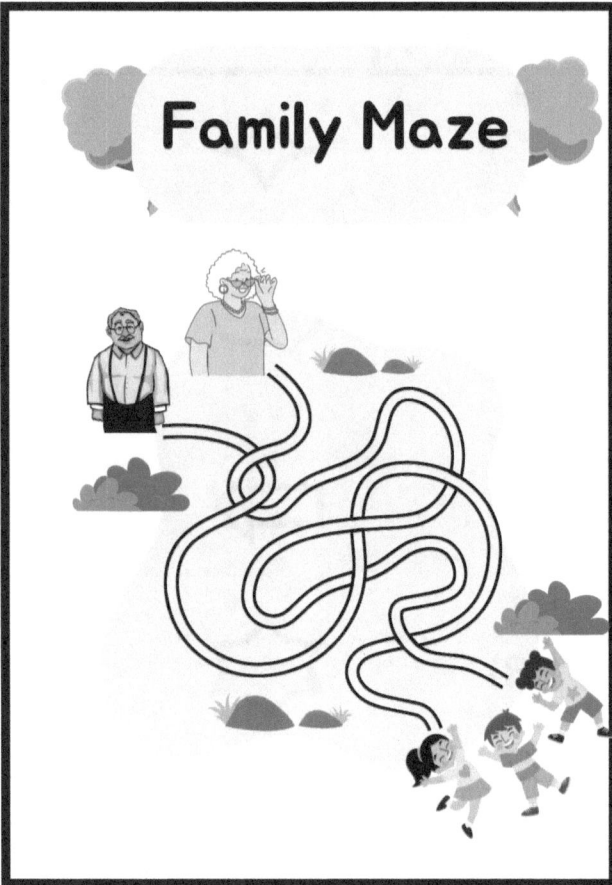

Emergency Workers Maze

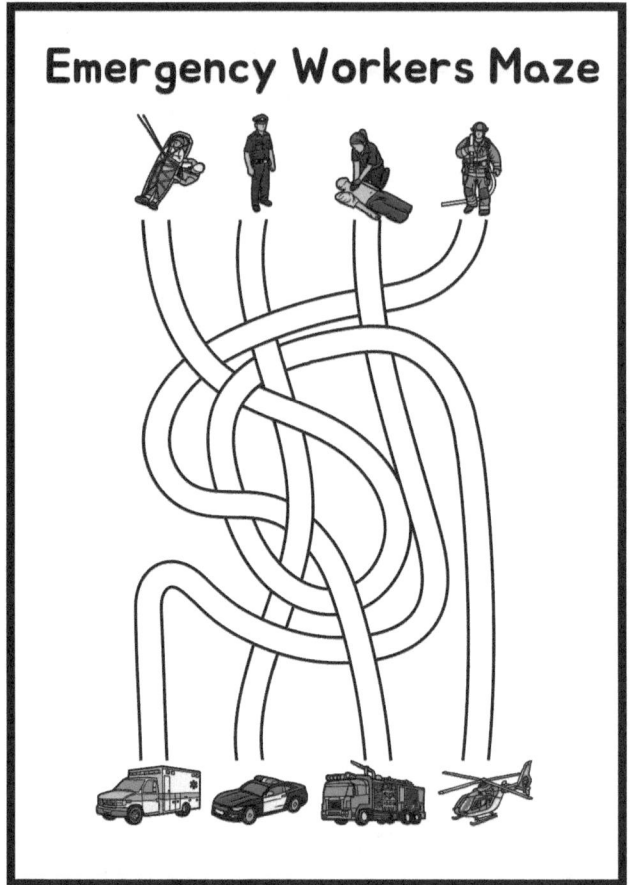

Jobs Maze
Different solutions

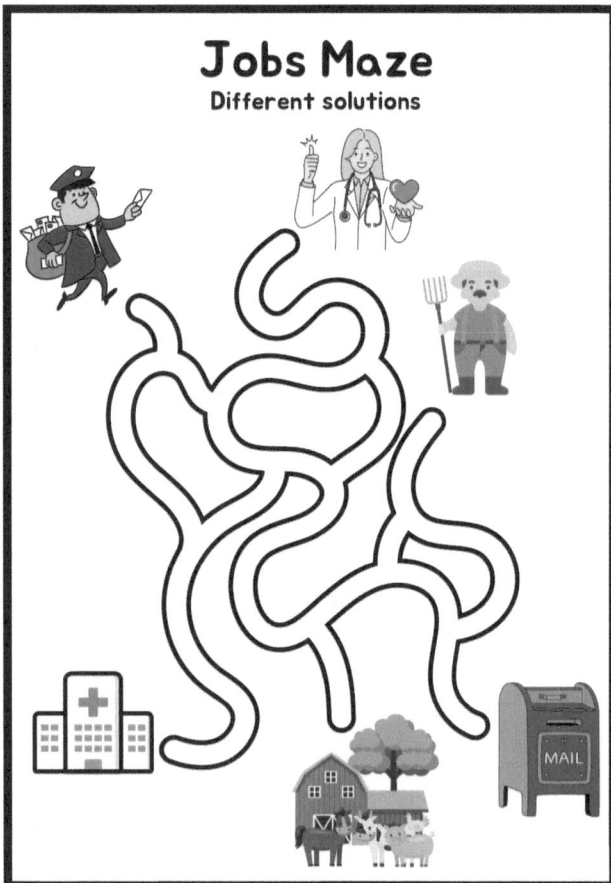

Recovery Maze
Different solutions

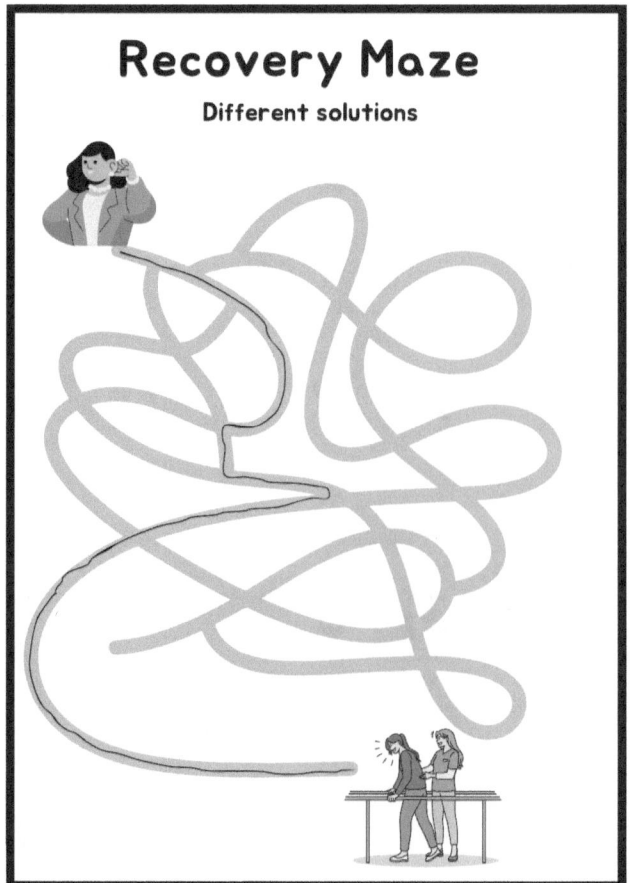

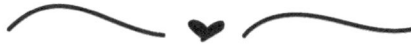

Unlock Your Free Bonus Content!

Scan the **QR code** to access exclusive bonus content for free! You can also request access by emailing us at:

hello@vitalstepsbooks.com

Don't miss out on these valuable extras to enhance your experience!

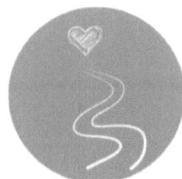

Vital Steps Books

Memory Skills

★ **Usefulness:**

Enhanced Recall Abilities

Increased Retention of New Information

Improved Cognitive Resilience

Greater Independence in Daily Activities

INSTRUCTIONS

📌 It is advised not to use a highlighter as it could bleed through the page.

📌 In some statements, the explanation of the exercise is highlighted. In these cases, it involves an additional task to be performed to increase the difficulty of the exercise.

📌 The solutions are found at the end of each section.

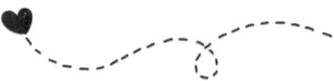

Memorize the positions of the CLOCK. Try to indicate in the box on page 81 the position you remember.

Between both pages, there is a counting exercise, which you can do to increase the difficulty of the activity.

Find This Object

Could you find **FIVE SPATULAS** in this picture?

Do you remember?

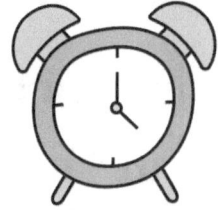

Memorize the positions of the HAT. Try to indicate in the box on page 84 the position you remember. Between both pages, there is a counting exercise, which you can do to increase the difficulty of the activity.

Find This Object

Could you find SIX CUPS in this picture?

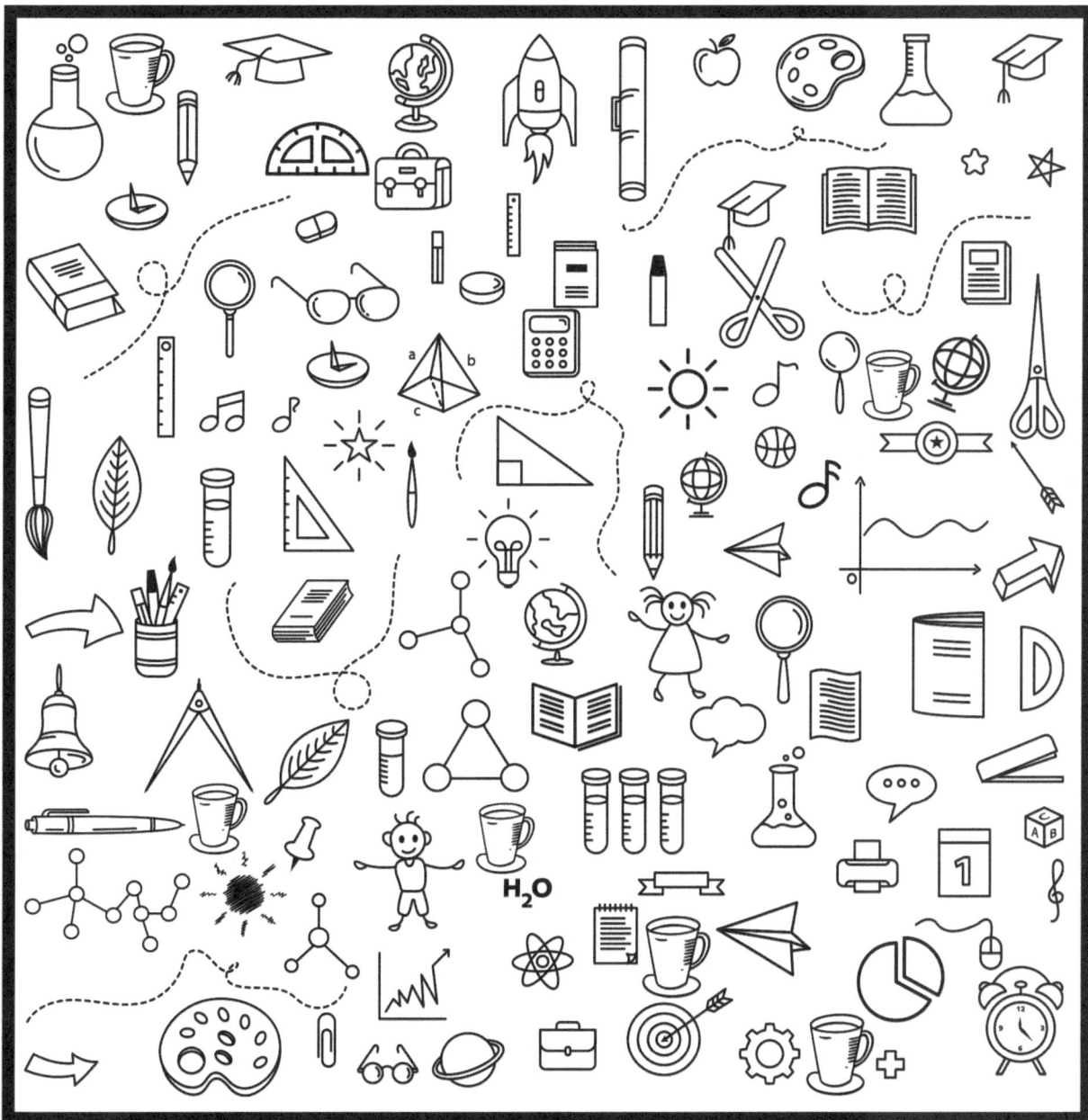

Do you remember?

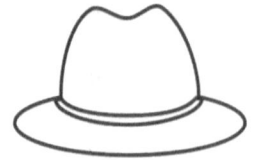

Memorize the positions of the PHONE. Try to indicate in the box on page 87 the position you remember.

Between both pages, there is a counting exercise, which you can do to increase the difficulty of the activity.

Find This Object

Could you find FIVE SCREWS in this picture?

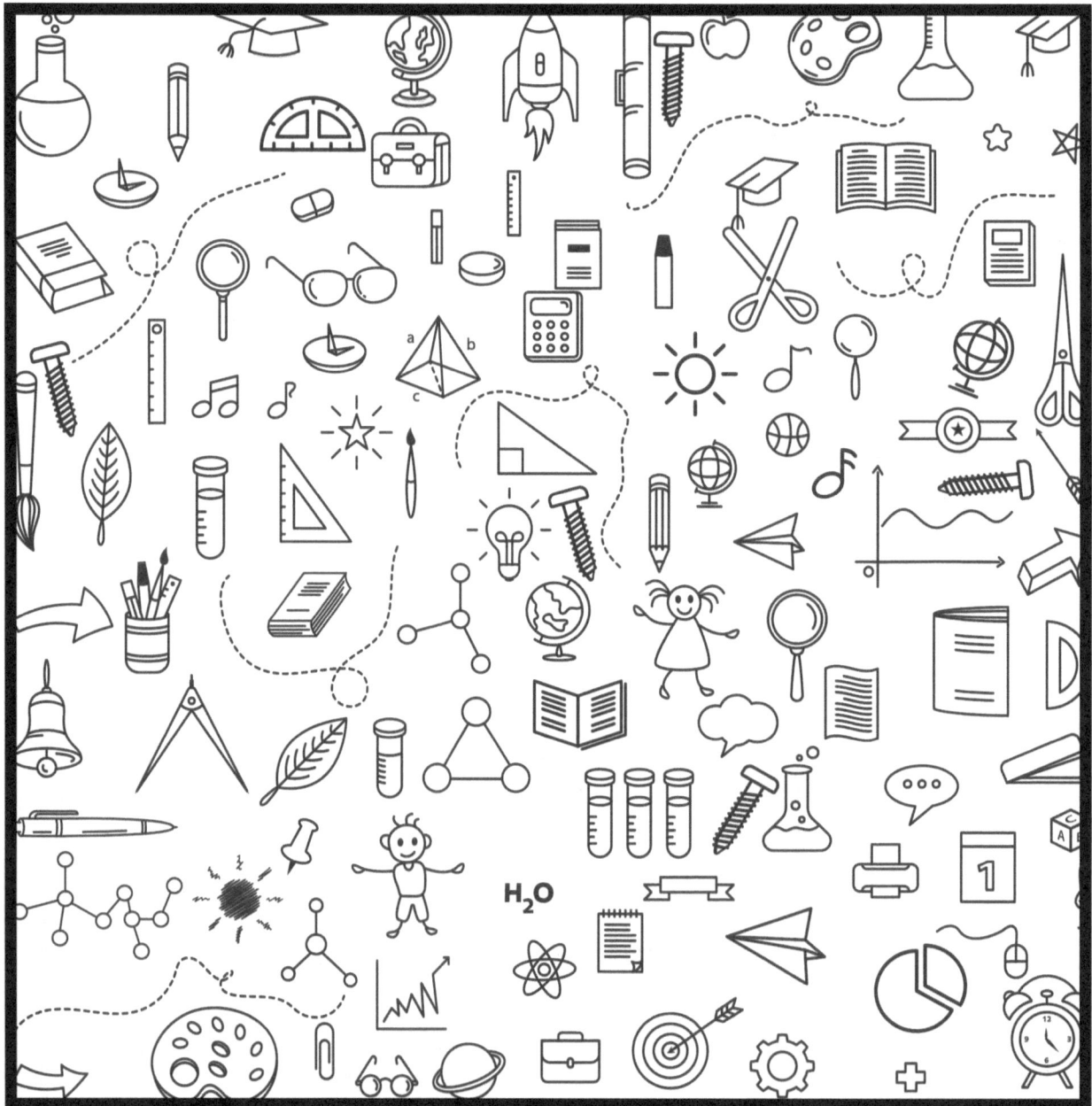

Do you remember?

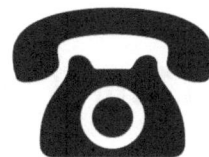

Memorize the positions of the BOOK. Try to indicate in the box on page 90 the position you remember. Between both pages, there is a counting exercise, which you can do to increase the difficulty of the activity.

Find This Object

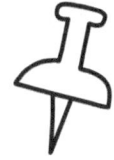

Could you find FIVE PINS in this picture?

Do you remember?

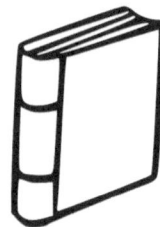

Observe and memorize the following images. Try to locate them in the grid on page 93.

Between both pages, there is a counting exercise, which you can perform to increase the difficulty of the activity.

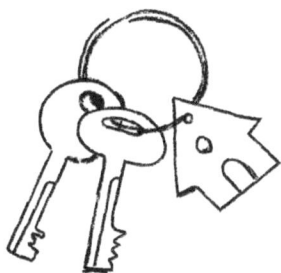

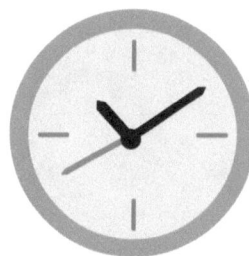

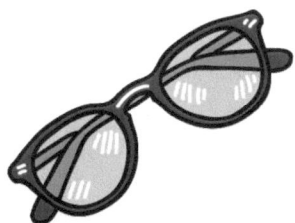

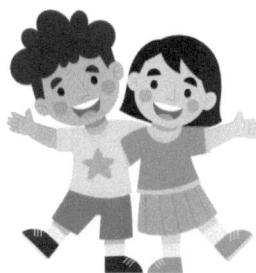

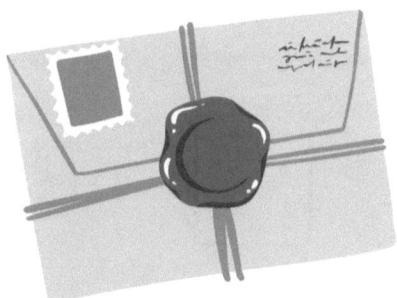

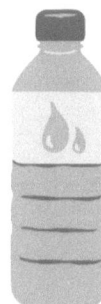

Let's Count in Spring

Count and write your answers in the chart below

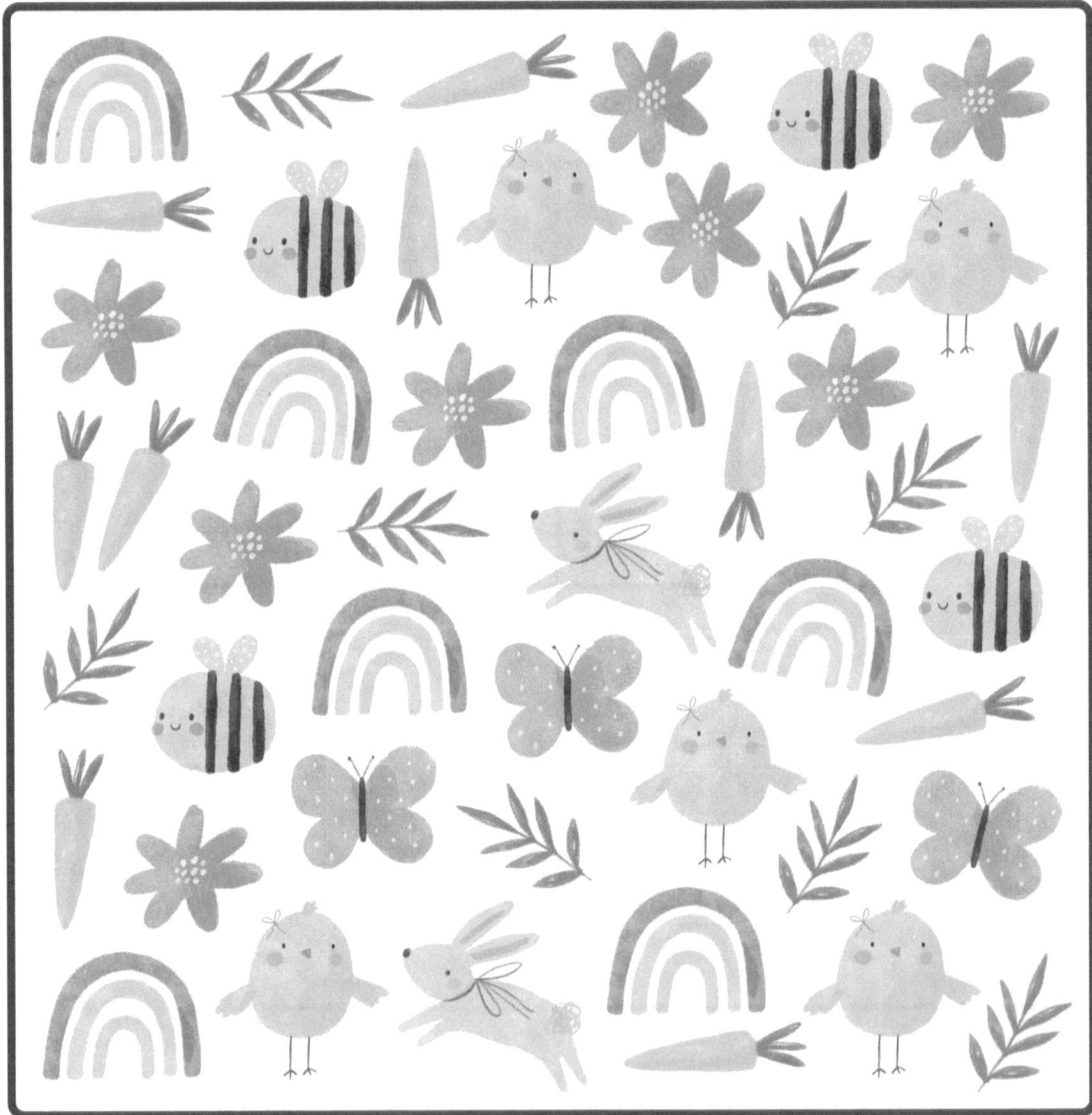

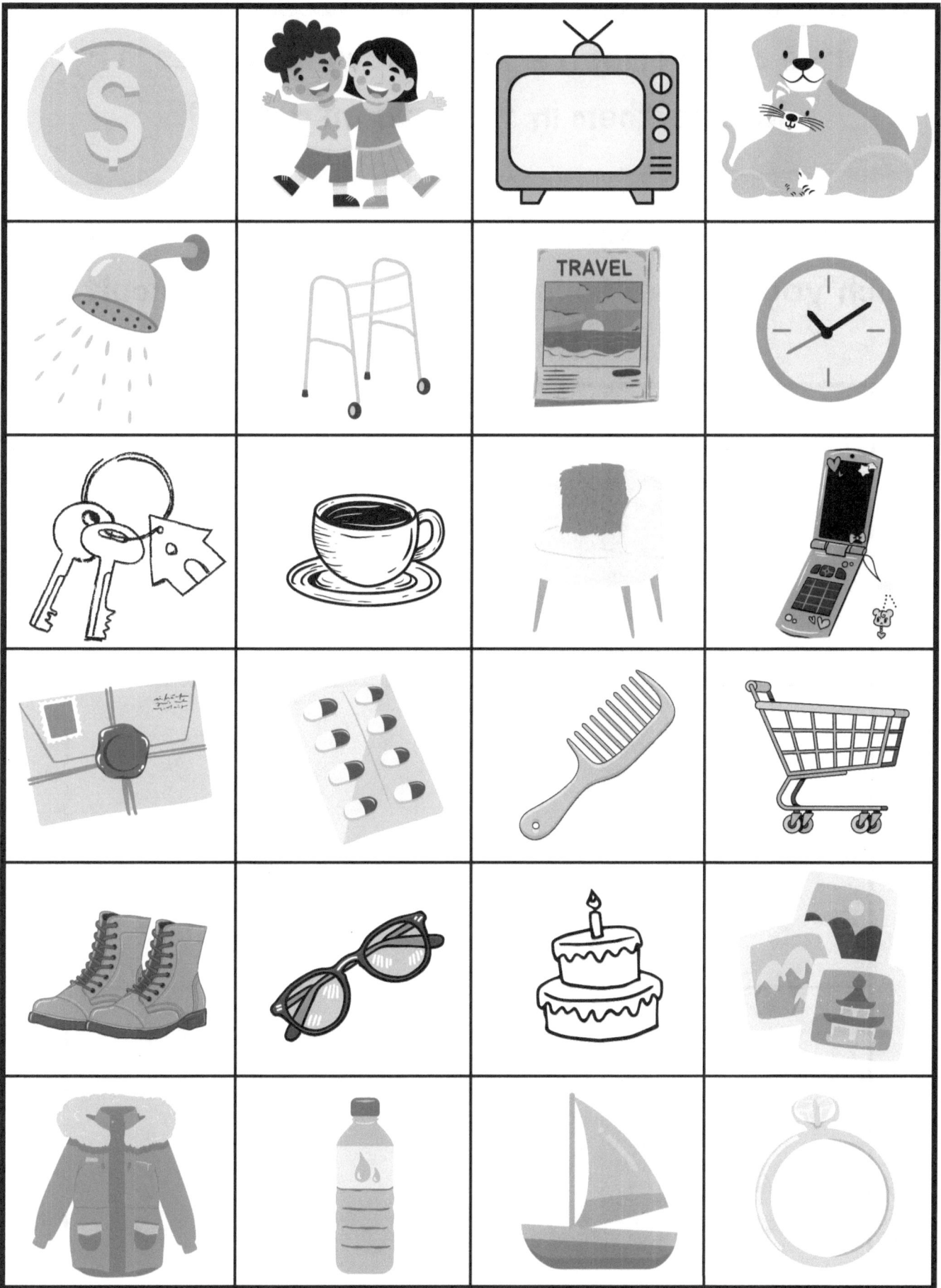

Observe and memorize the following images. Try to locate them in the grid on page 96.

Between both pages, there is a counting exercise, which you can perform to increase the difficulty of the activity.

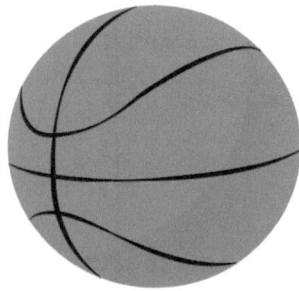

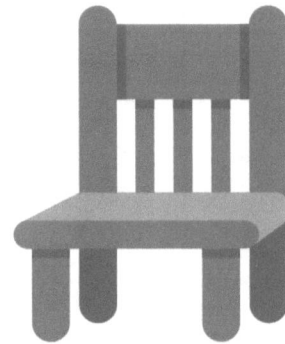

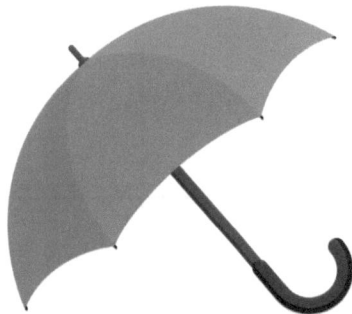

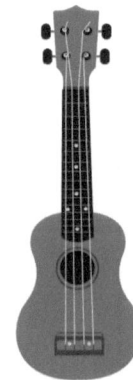

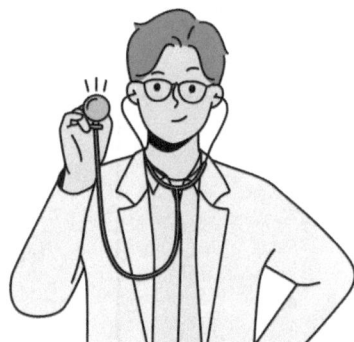

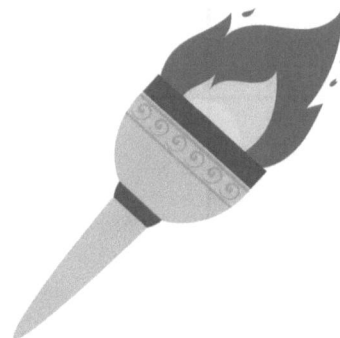

Let's Count Pets

Count and write your answers in the chart below

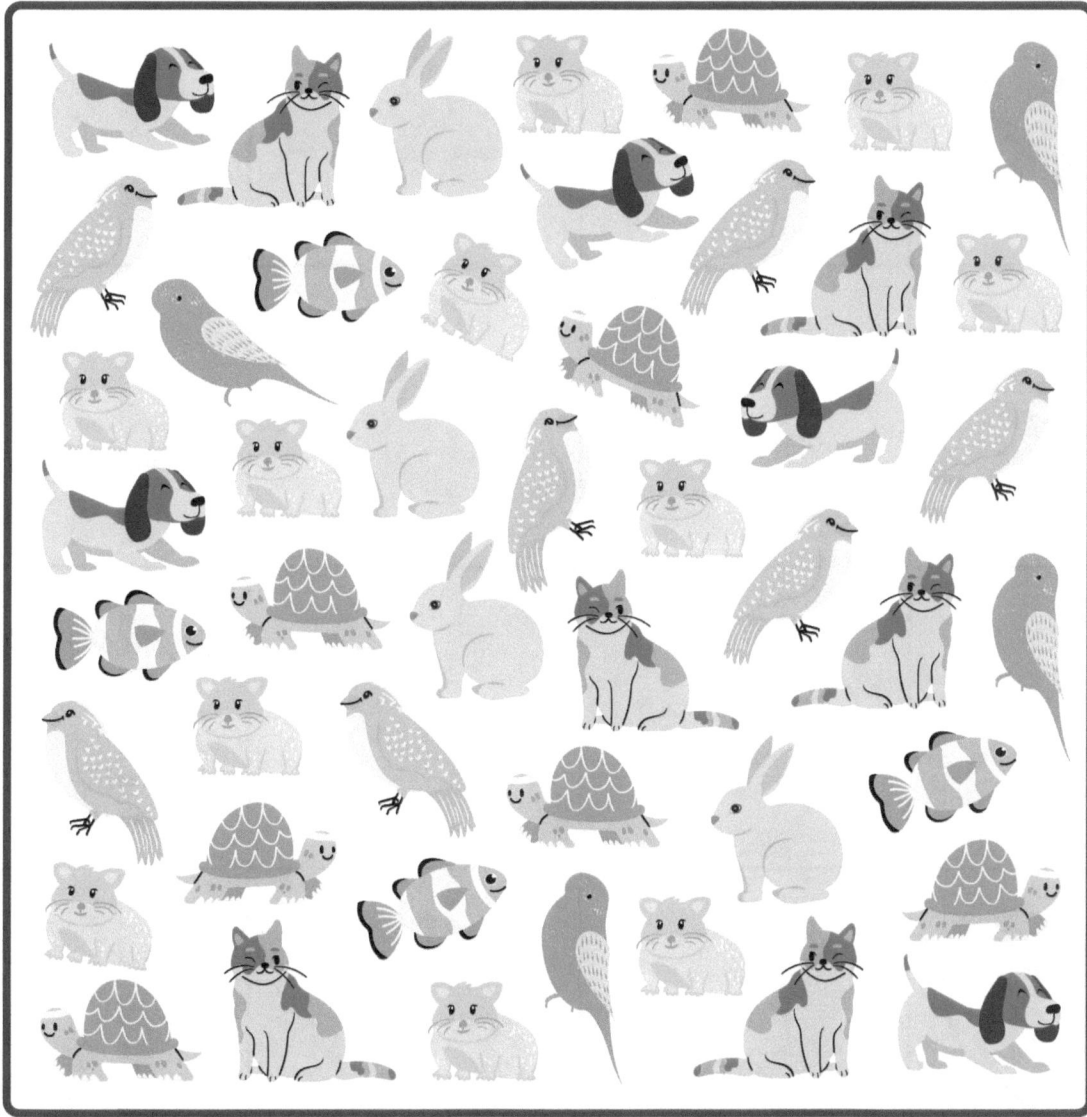

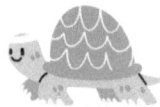

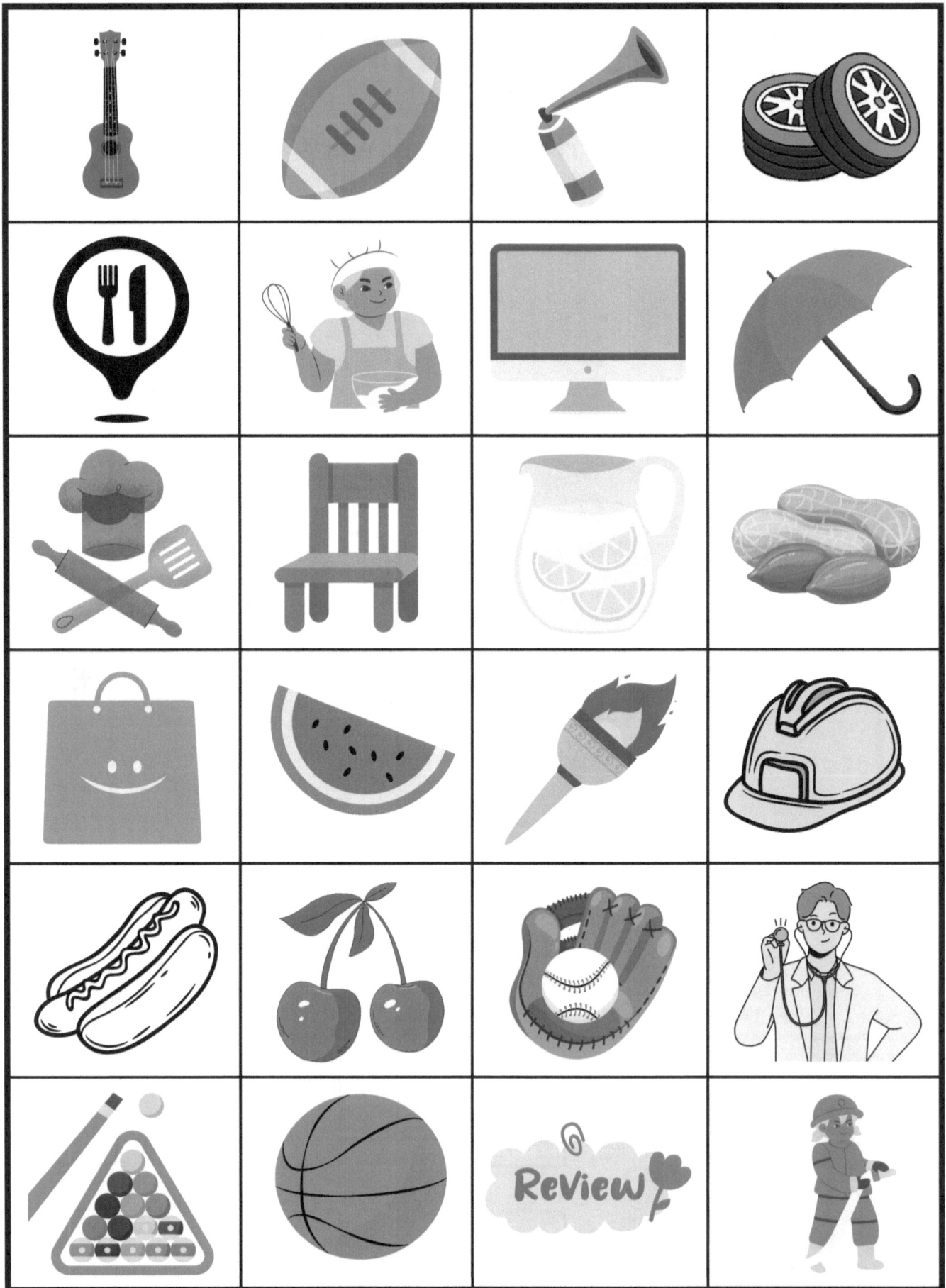

Observe and memorize the following images. Try to locate them in the grid on page 99.

Between both pages, there is a counting exercise, which you can perform to increase the difficulty of the activity.

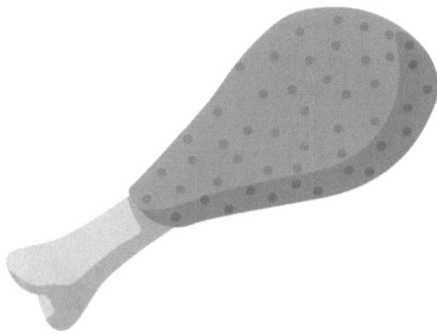

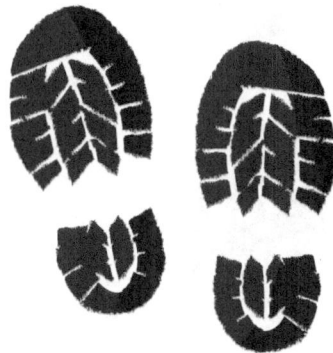

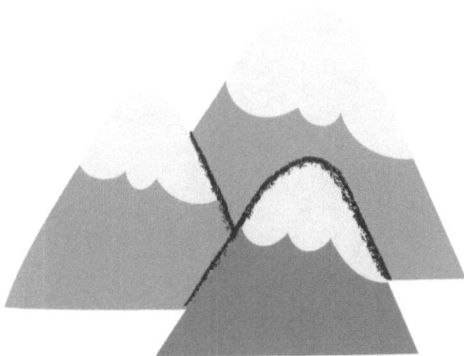

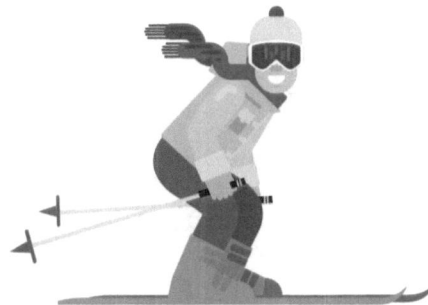

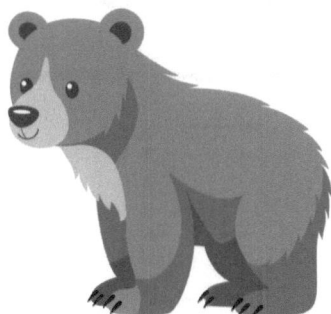

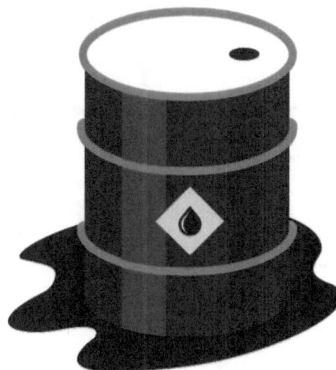

Let's Count Ocean Animals

Count and write your answers in the chart below

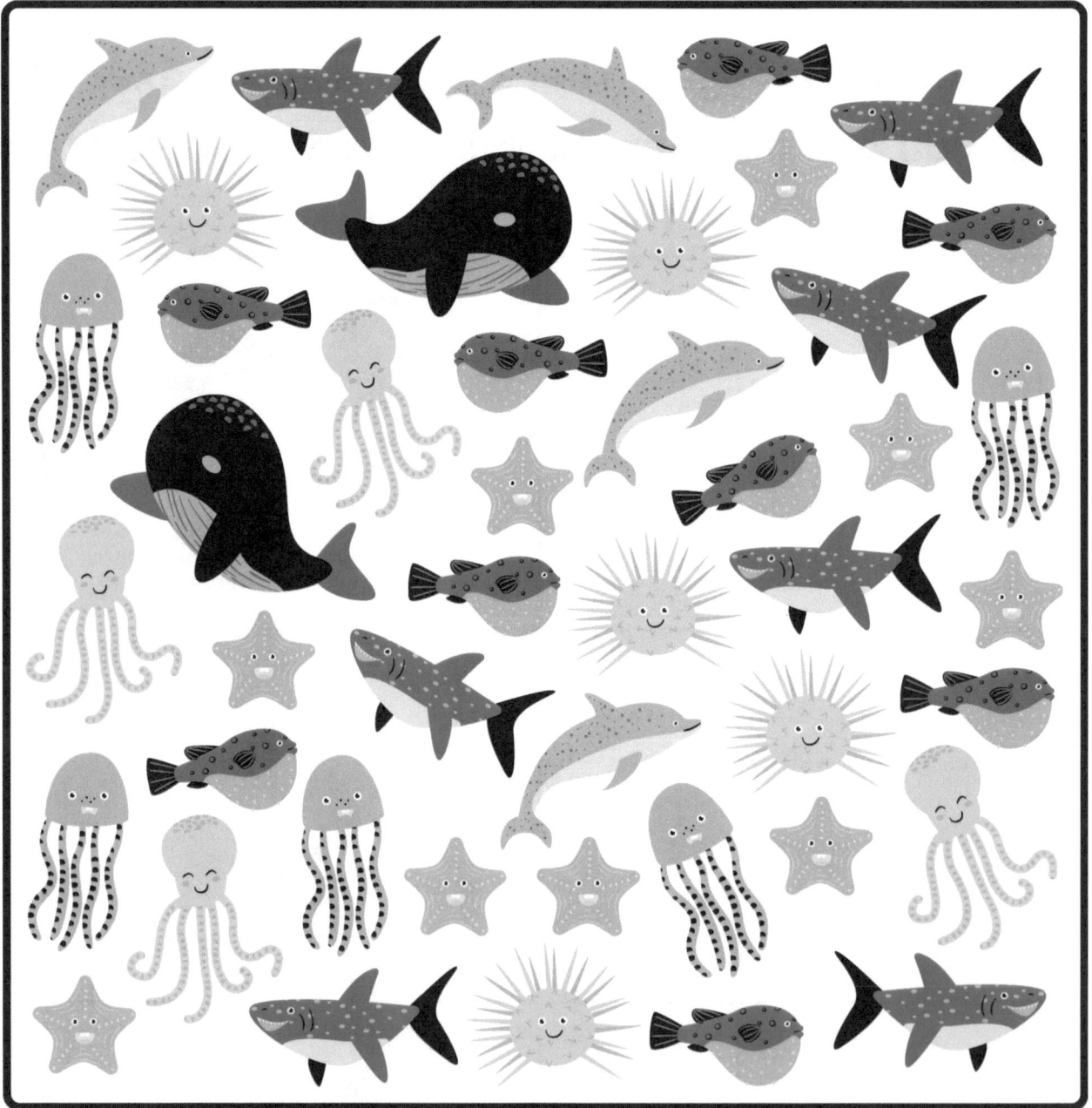

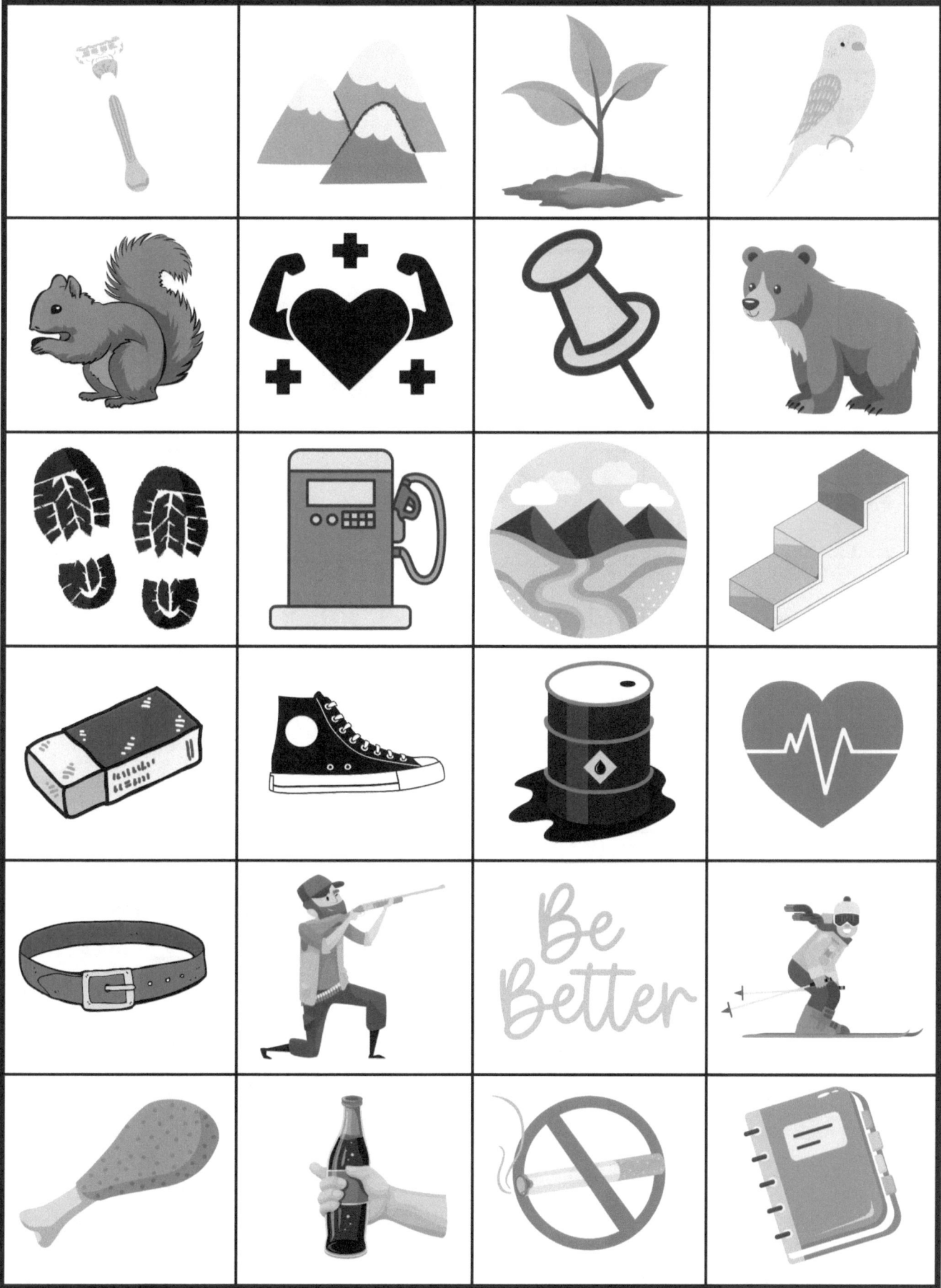

Family Crossword Puzzle

Try to fill in the crossword with the clues provided in the box below.

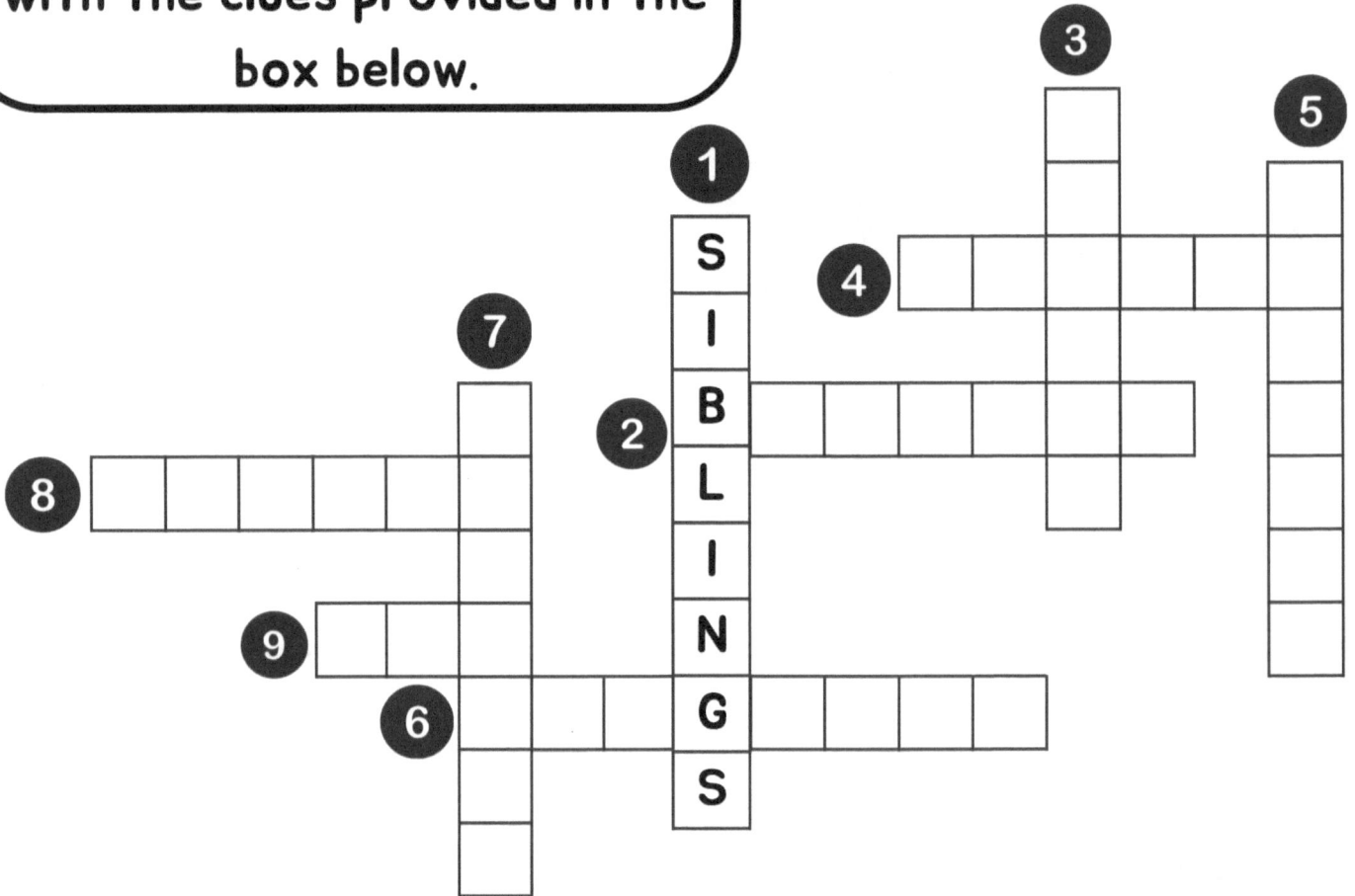

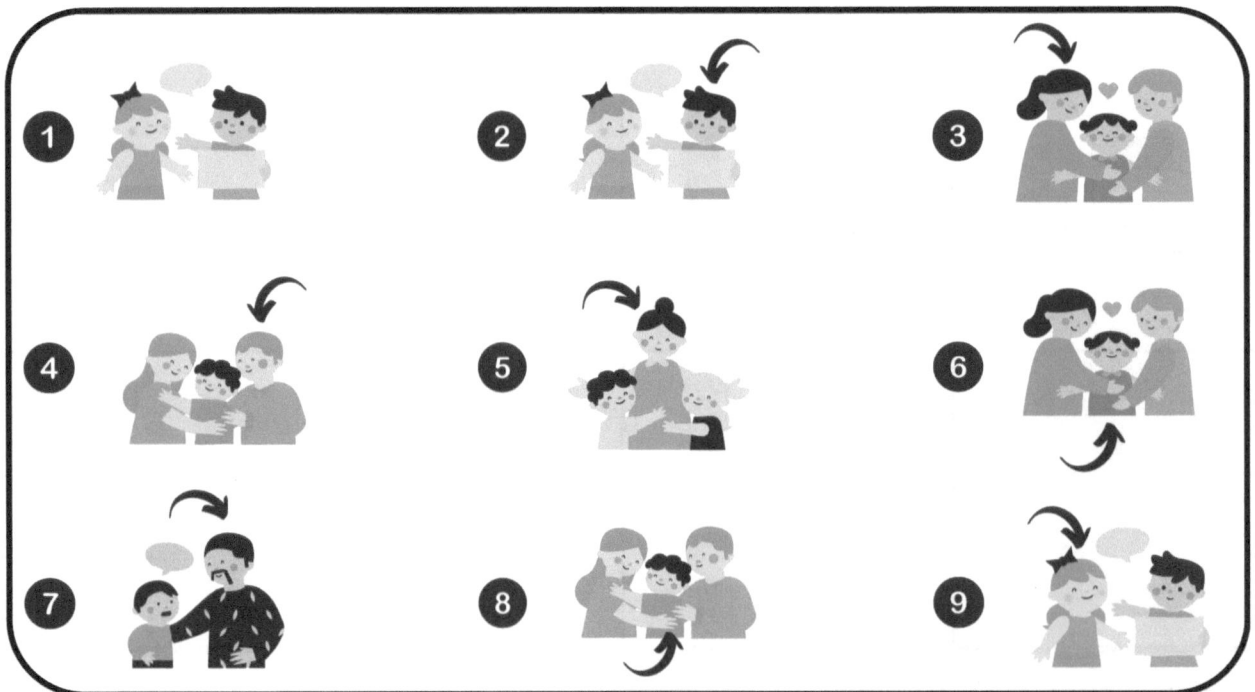

1 Down: SIBLINGS

100

Keys

Spatulas

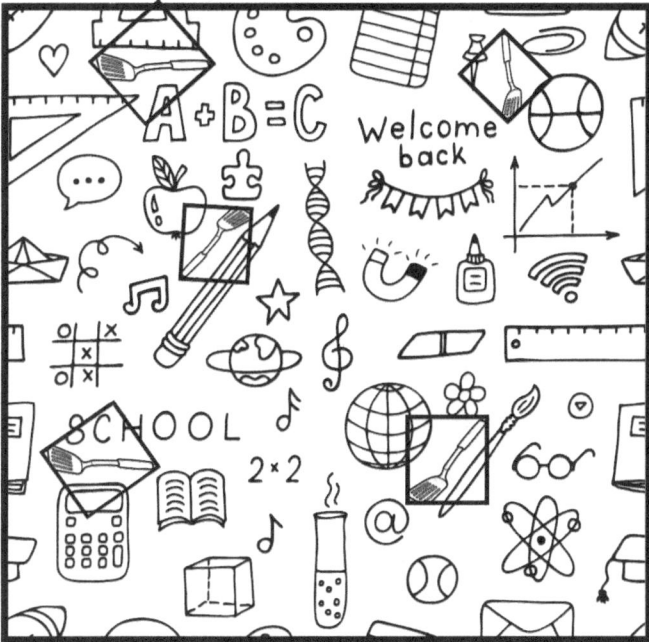

Cups

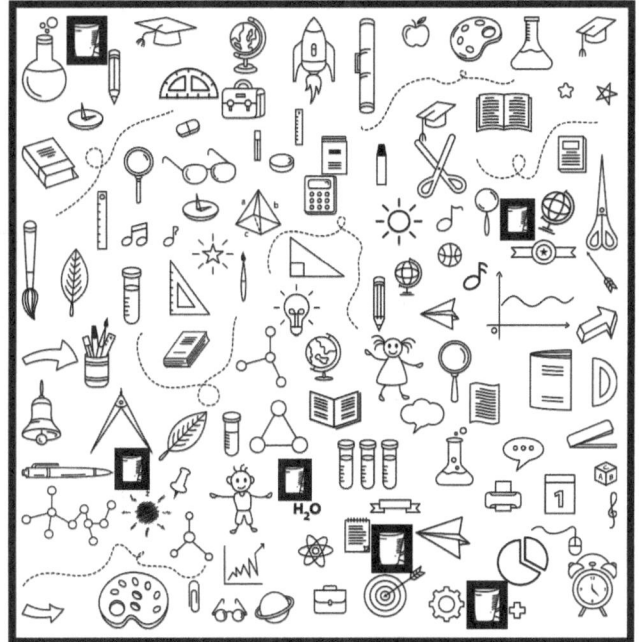

Screws

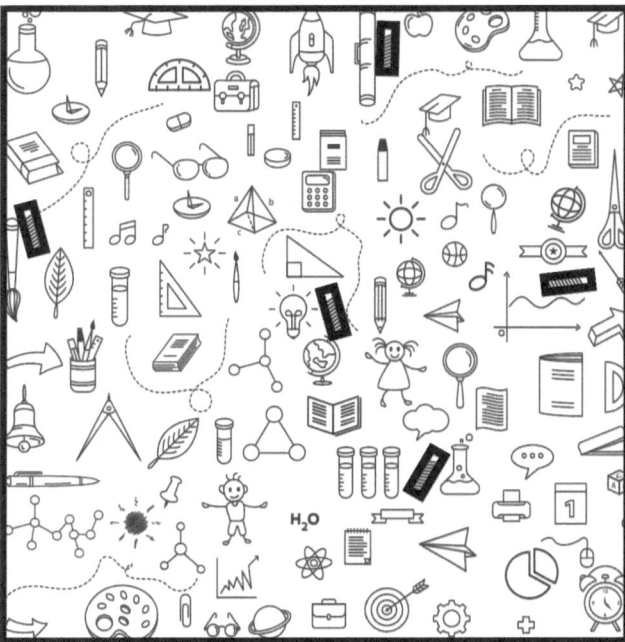

Pins

Keys

rainbow	7	chick	5	butterfly	3	leaf	8
flower	8	rabbit	2	bee	4	carrot	10

- -

dog	5	hamster	11	cat	6	budgie	4
clownfish	4	turtle	7	rabbit	4	parrot	7

- -

whale	2	octopus	4	jellyfish	5	starfish	9
shark	7	urchin	5	dolphin	4	pufferfish	9

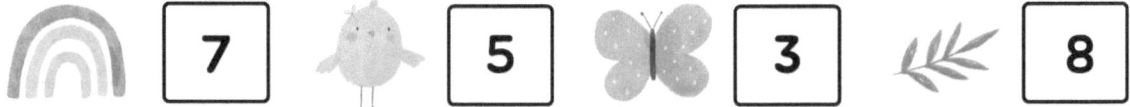

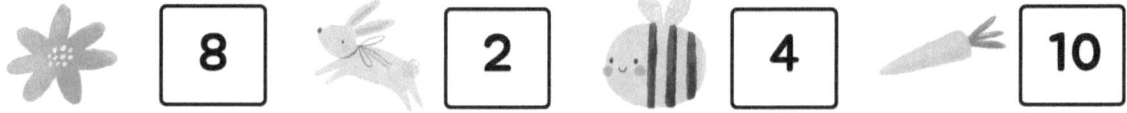

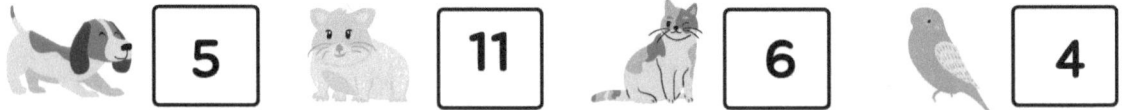

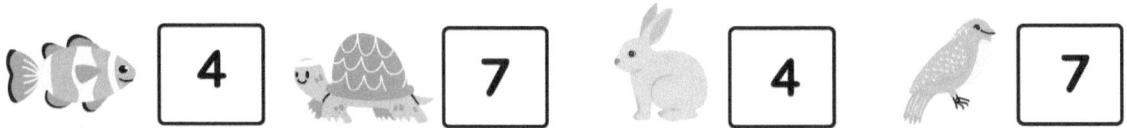

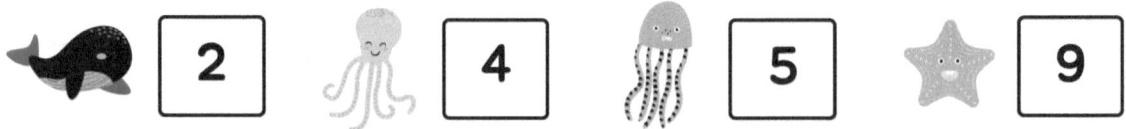

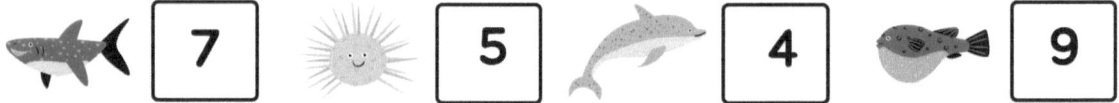

Family Crossword Puzzle

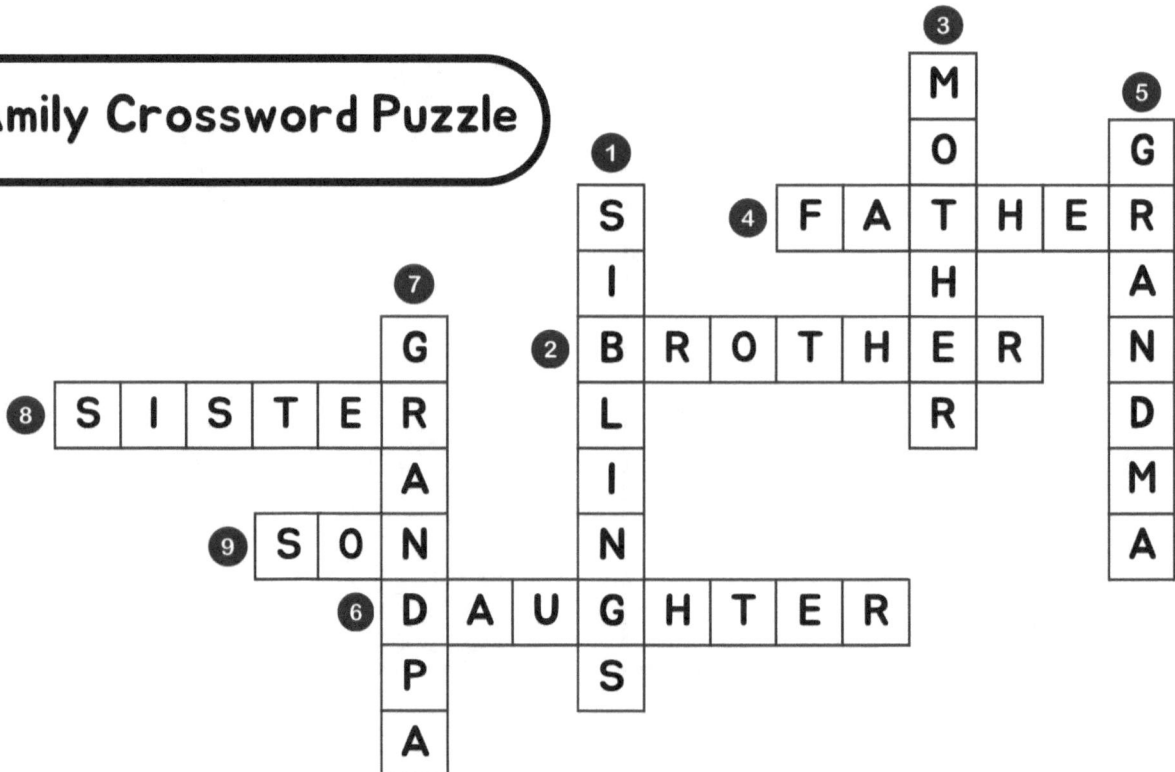

```
                                    ³M
                                     O
        ¹S              ⁴F A T H E R      ⁵G
         I                   H            R
    ⁷G  ²B R O T H E R       E            A
⁸S I S T E R                 R            N
    R   L                                 D
    A  ²S O N                              M
    N   I                                 A
  ⁹S O N N
  ⁶D A U G H T E R
    P   S
    A
```

102

Communication Skills

-Naming

-Reading Comprehension

-Sentence Formation

★ **Usefulness:**

Improved Speech Clarity
Enhanced Language Comprehension
Expanded Vocabulary
Increased Social Interaction

INSTRUCTIONS

📌 It is advised not to use a highlighter as it could bleed through the page.

📌 In some statements, the explanation of the exercise is highlighted. In these cases, it involves an additional task to be performed to increase the difficulty of the exercise.

📌 The solutions are found at the end of each section.

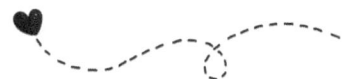

FIND THE WORD

Choose the letters to make the word from the box. Repeat the word and think about the last time you used it.

B   A

U   T

C 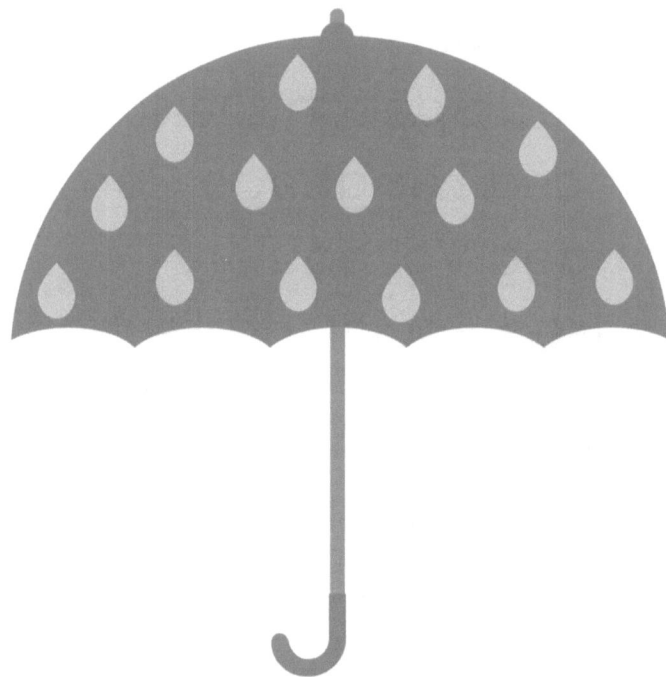 C

M   L

Z   Z

UMBRELLA

I   S

B   L   R   T   E   L

FIND THE WORD

Choose the letters to make the word from the box. Repeat the word and think about which one is your favorite and why.

D   A

U   T

J   C

M   L

Z   E

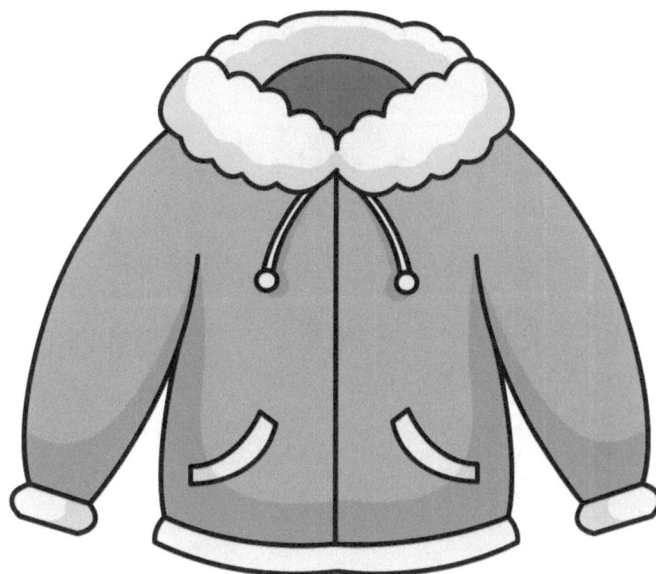

JACKET

I   S

A   L   R   C   K   L

FIND THE WORD

Choose the letters to make the word from the box. Repeat the word and think about which ones are more comfortable.

S   I

A   S

F   C

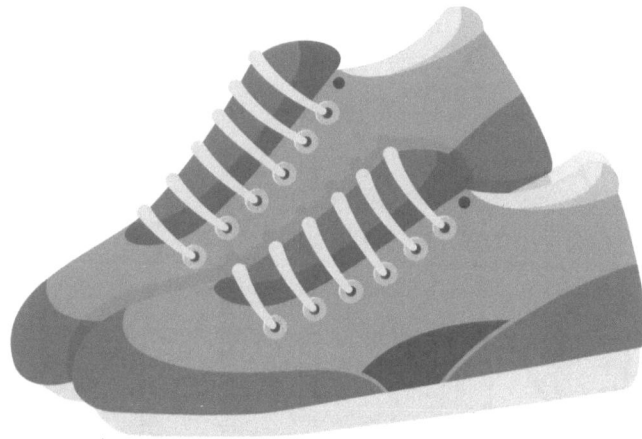

H   T

Z   N

SHOES

L   E

P   O   W   R   K   L

Reading Comprehension

Read the sentence inside the box and choose the object that is most related.

a) Used in the hospital

b) Used in recovery activities

Reading Comprehension

Read the sentence inside the box and choose the object that is most related.

c) **Used to be on time**

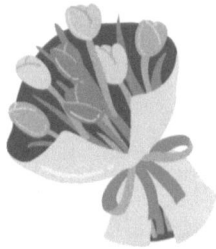

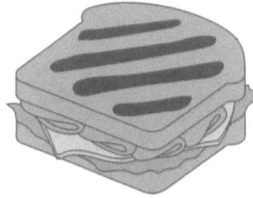

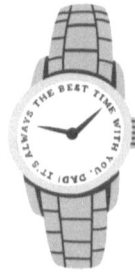

d) **Used to talk with my family**

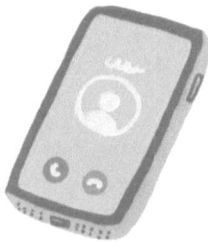

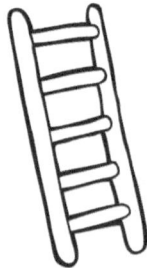

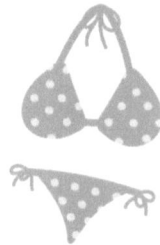

Reading Comprehension

Read the sentence inside the box and choose the object that is most related.

e)

Used to open the door

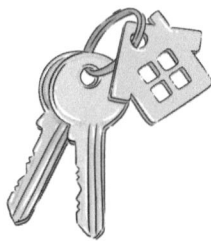

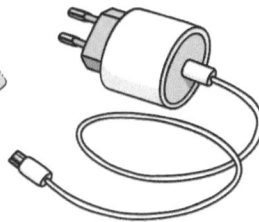

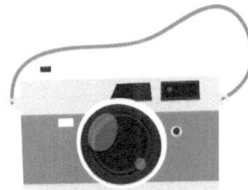

f)

Used to pay in a store

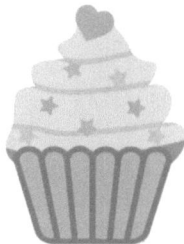

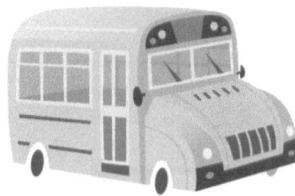

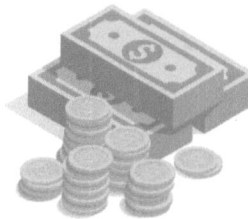

Nomination - 1

Look at the object and write the name to the right.

<u>Try to pronounce the words.</u>

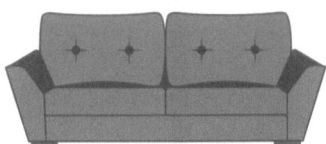 ⟶

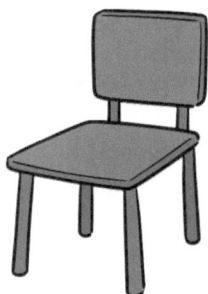 ⟶

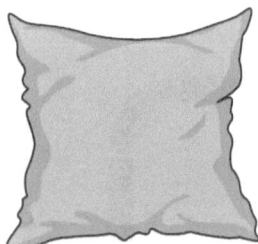 ⟶

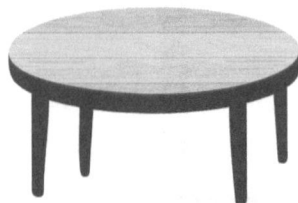 ⟶

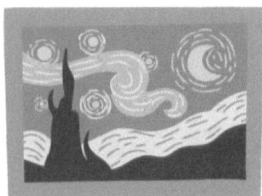 ⟶

Nomination - 2

Look at the object and write the name to the right.

Try to describe the image.

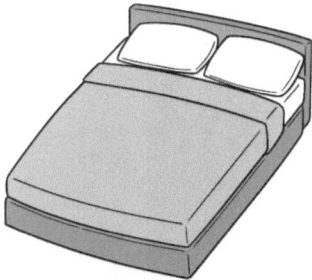

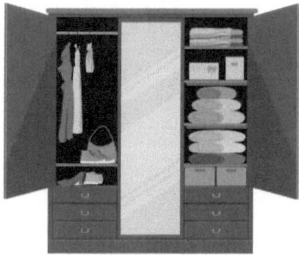

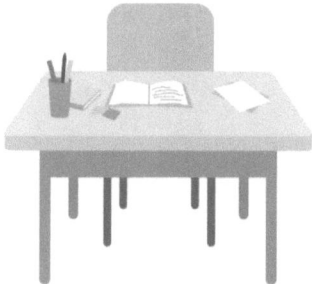

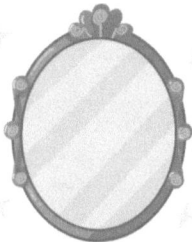

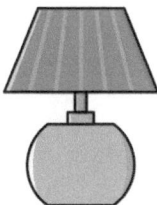

Nomination - 3

Look at the object and write the name to the right.

Try to describe the utility of these objects.

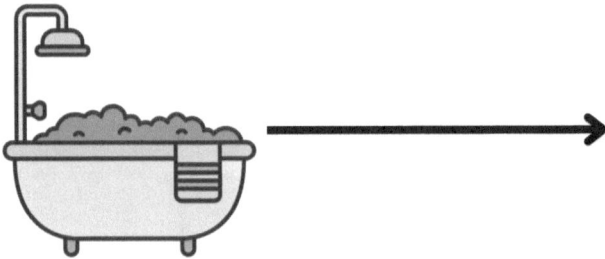 →

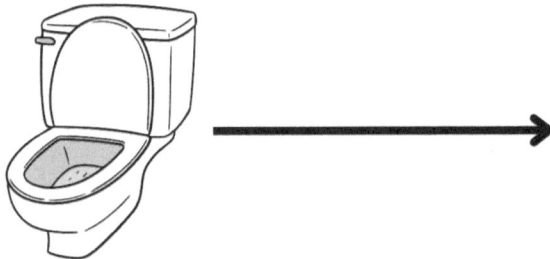 →

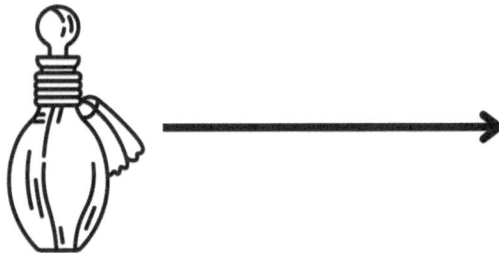 →

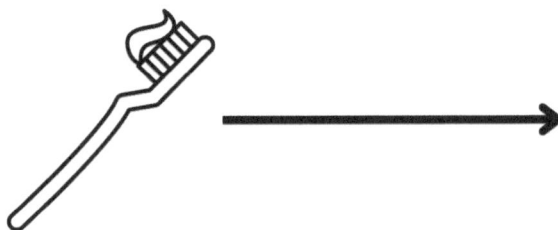 →

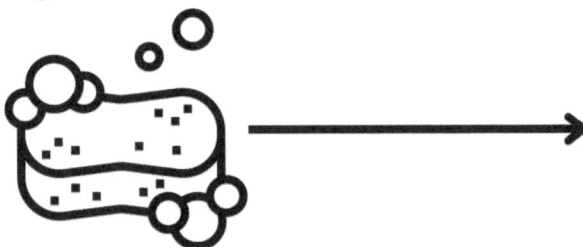 →

Nomination - 4

Look at the object and write the name to the right.

Try to repeat the words.

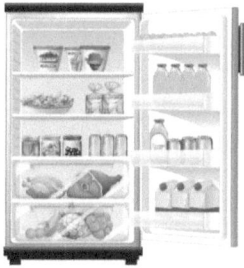

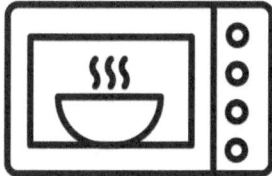

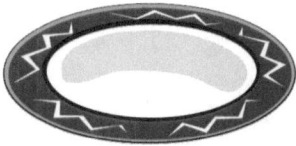

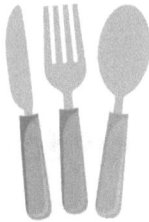

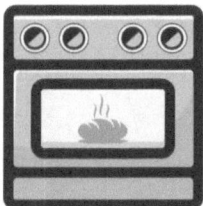

Category - 1

Observe the following pictures. Write the name of each object in the column of the category it belongs to. <u>Explain why it corresponds to that category.</u>

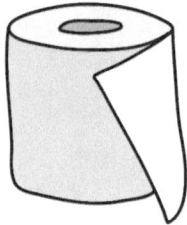

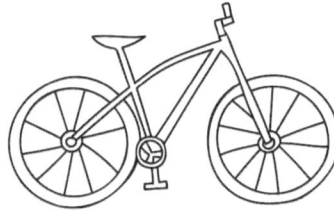

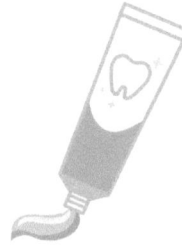

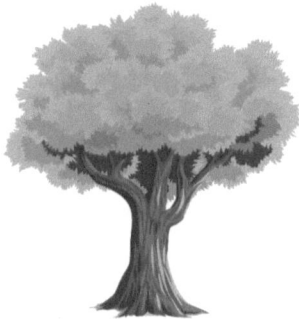

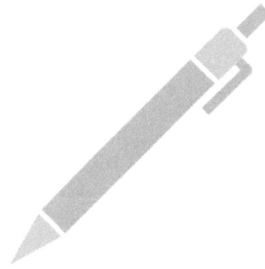

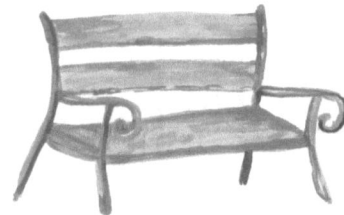

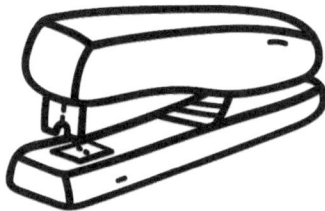

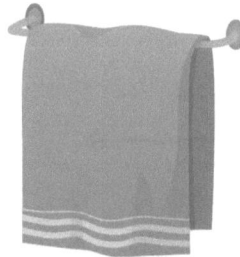

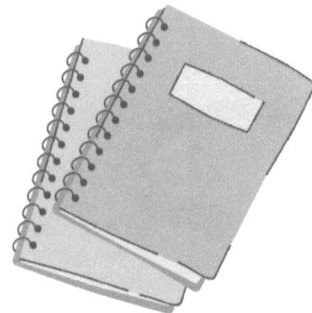

Bathroom	Office	Outdoor
. . . .	. . . .	. . . .
. . . .	. . . .	. . . .
. . . .	. . . .	. . . .

Category - 2

Observe the following pictures. Write the name of each object in the column of the category it belongs to. _Explain in your own words your experience with these objects._

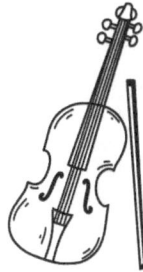

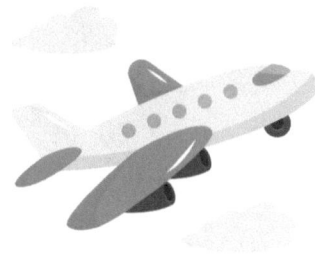

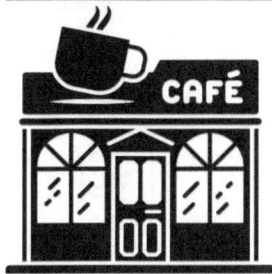

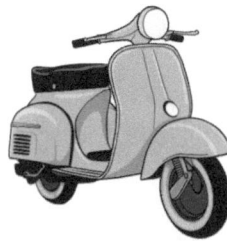

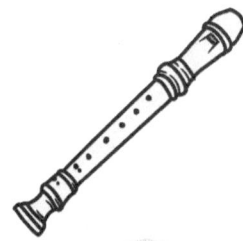

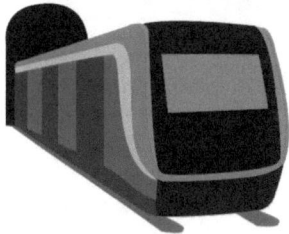

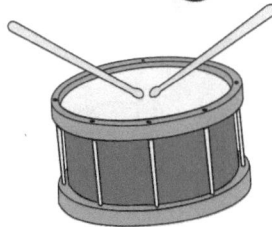

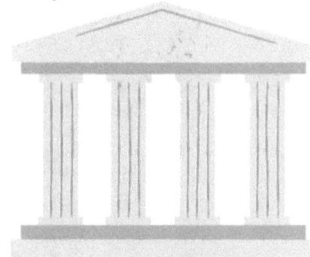

Musical Instruments	Transportation	Public Places
. . . .	. . . .	. . . .
. . . .	. . . .	. . . .
. . . .	. . . .	. . . .

Category - 3

Observe the following pictures. Write the name of each object in the column of the category it belongs to. **Think of more related objects and pronounce them.**

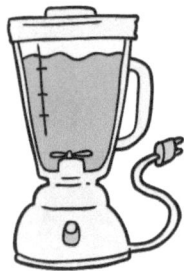

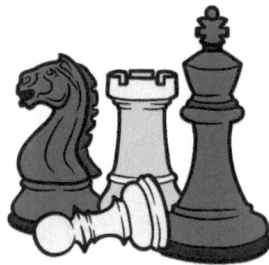

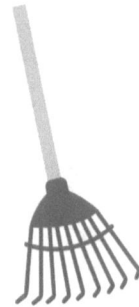

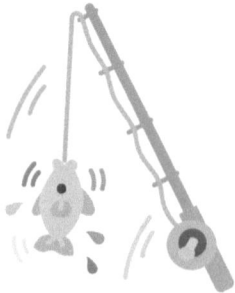

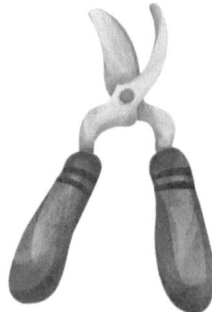

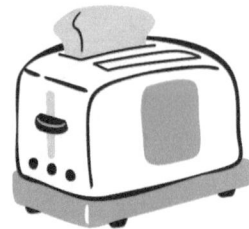

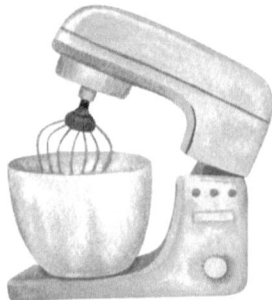

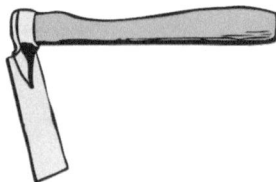

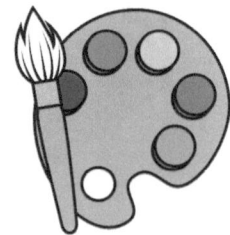

Leisure Activities	Gardening Tools	Kitchen Appliances
. . . .	. . . .	. . . .
. . . .	. . . .	. . . .
. . . .	. . . .	. . . .

Sentence Building - 1

Arrange the words to form sentences. Write the correct sentences on the lines.

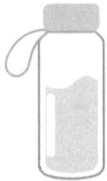 | water. | Drink | cool | some

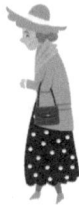 | a | walk. | Take | short

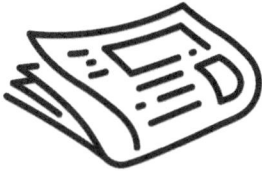 | the | paper. | morning | Read

 | hot. | The | sun | is

<u>Hint</u>: the word that begins with a capital letter occupies the first position. The word that is followed by a full stop occupies the last position.

Sentence Building - 2

Arrange the words to form sentences. Write the correct sentences on the lines.

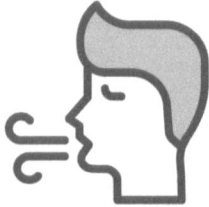 | deeply | relax. | and | Breathe |

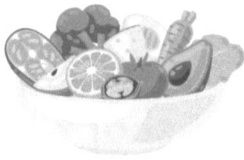 | a | Eat | meal. | healthy |

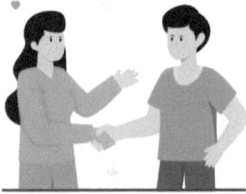 | Greet | friend. | close | a |

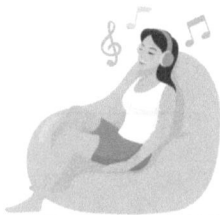 | to | The | music. | soothing |

<u>Hint</u>: the word that begins with a capital letter occupies the first position. The word that is followed by a full stop occupies the last position.

Sentence Building - 3

Arrange the words to form sentences. Write the correct sentences on the lines.

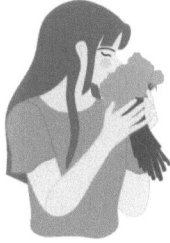 | Smell | flowers | fresh | the |

_____

- -

_____

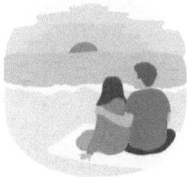 | high | up | arms | Stretch |

_____

- -

_____

| calmy | sunset | Watch | the |

_____

- -

_____

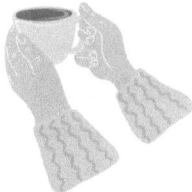 | cup | Hold | warm | the |

_____

- -

_____

<u>Hint</u>: the word that begins with a capital letter occupies the first position.

Keys

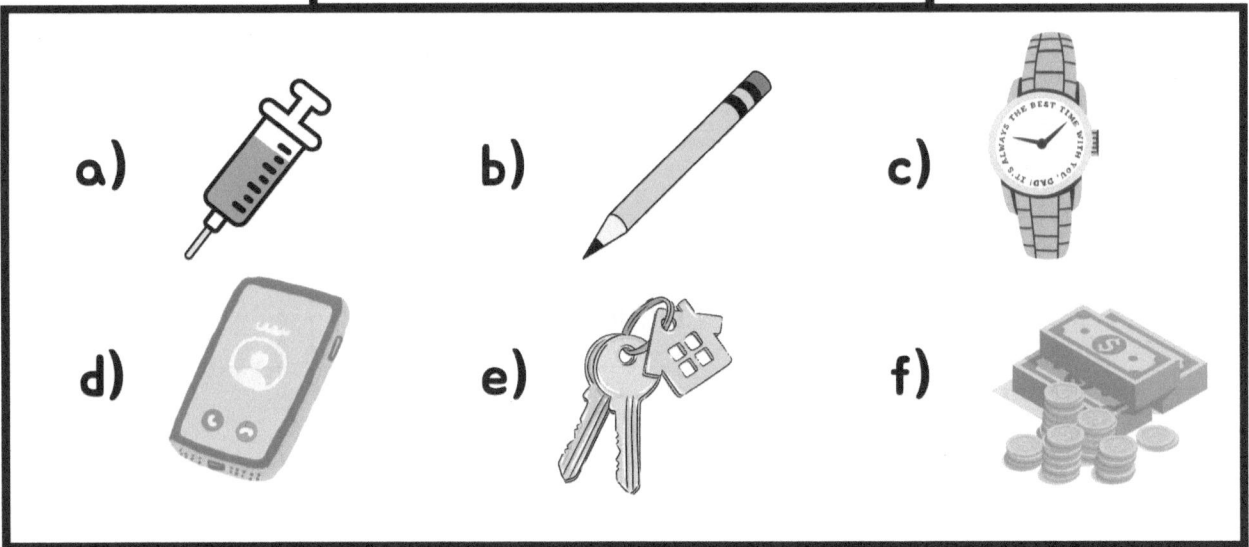

a) b) c)

d) e) f)

Nomination 1

- Sofa, couch,
- Chair
- Cushion, pillow
- Table
- Picture

Nomination 2

- Bed
- Cupboard, wardrobe
- Desk
- Mirror
- Lamp

Nomination 3

- Bathtub, tub, bath
- Toilet
- Fragance, perfume
- Toothbrush
- Sponge

Nomination 4

- Fridge, refrigerator
- Microwave
- Dish, plate
- Cutlery
- Oven

Keys

Category 1		
Bathroom	**Office**	**Outdoor**
Toilet paper	Pen	Bicycle
Toothpaste	Stapler	Tree
Towel	Notebook	Bench

Category 2		
Musical Instruments	**Transportation**	**Public Places**
Violin	Scooter	Library
Drums	Subway	Coffee Shop, Cafe
Flute	Airplane	Museum

Category 3		
Leisure Activities	**Gardening Tools**	**Kitchen Apps.**
Chess	Hoe	Mixer
Painting	Rake	Toaster
Fishing	Shears	Blender

Keys

Sentence Building 1

"DRINK SOME COOL WATER."

"TAKE A SHORT WALK."

"READ THE MORNING PAPER."

"REST IN THE SHADE."

Sentence Building 2

"BREATHE DEEPLY AND RELAX."

"EAT A HEALTHY MEAL."

"GREET A CLOSE FRIEND."

"LISTEN TO SOOTHING MUSIC."

Sentence Building 3

"SMELL THE FRESH FLOWERS."

"STRETCH ARMS UP HIGH."

"WATCH THE SUNSET CALMLY."

"HOLD THE WARM CUP."

Fine Motor Skills

-Tracing

-Drawing and Coloring

★ **Usefulness:**
Enhanced Ability
Improved Hand-Eye Coordination
Increased Grip Strength
Better Precision

INSTRUCTIONS

📌 It is advised not to use a highlighter as it could bleed through the page.

📌 In some statements, the explanation of the exercise is highlighted. In these cases, it involves an additional task to be performed to increase the difficulty of the exercise.

📌 The solutions are found at the end of each section.

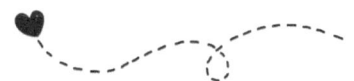

TRACE

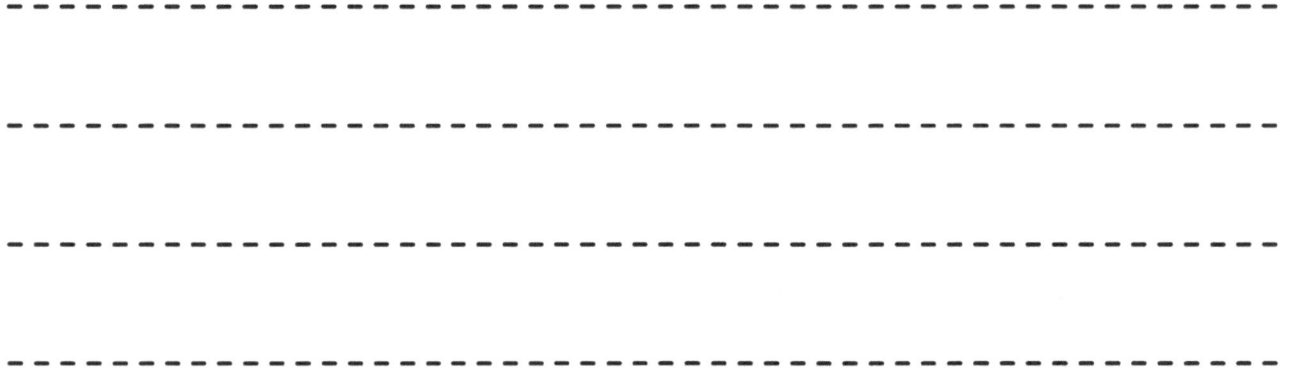

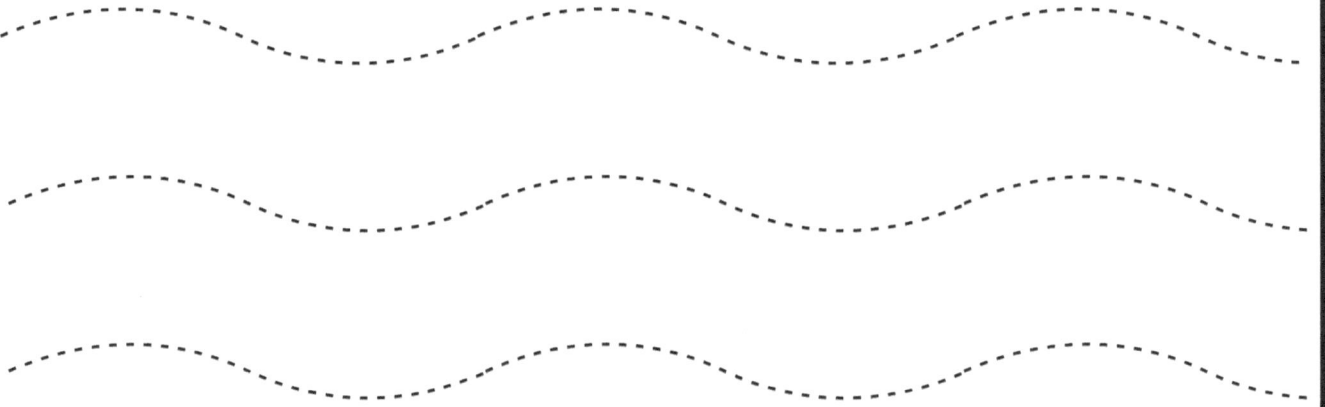

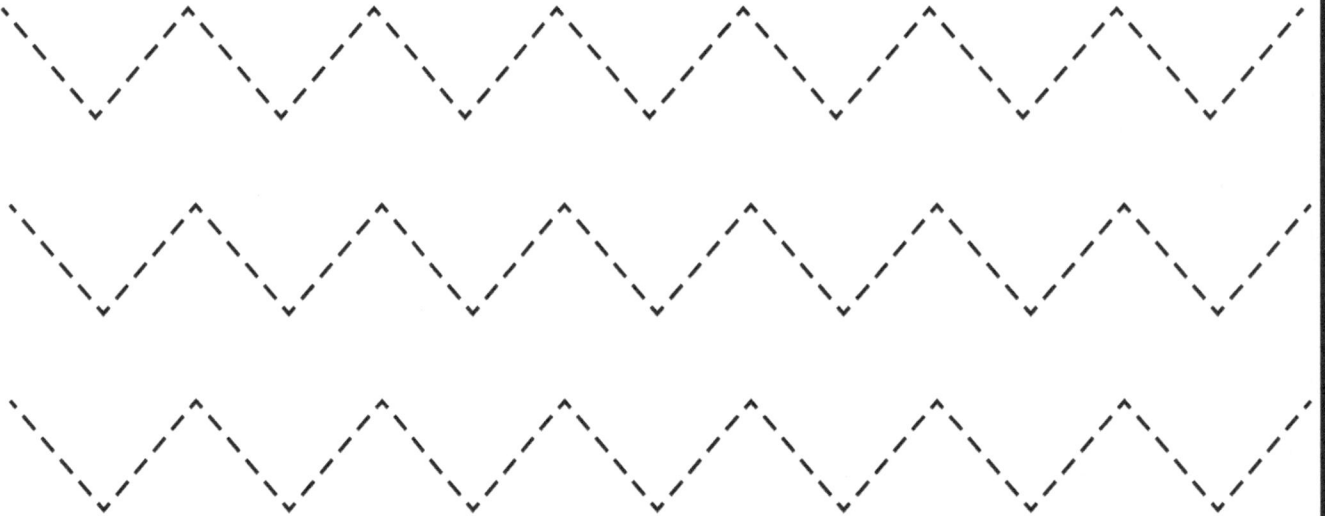

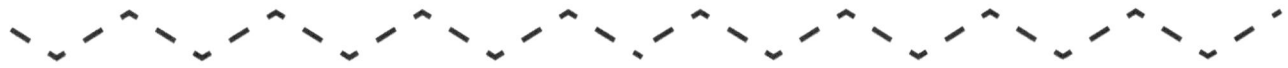

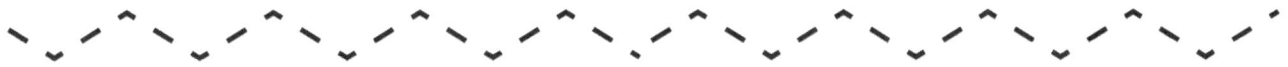

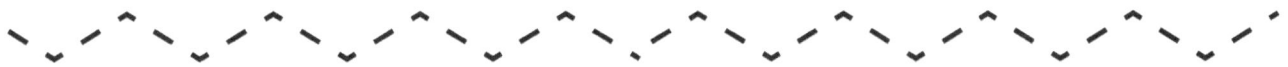

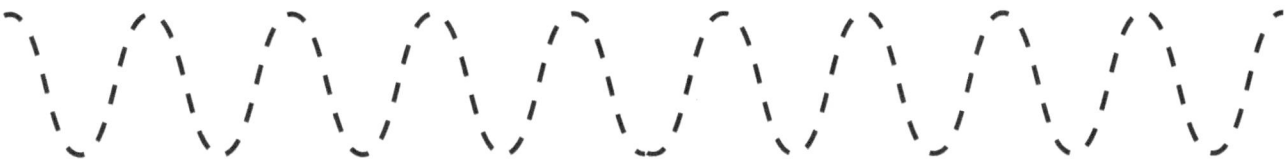

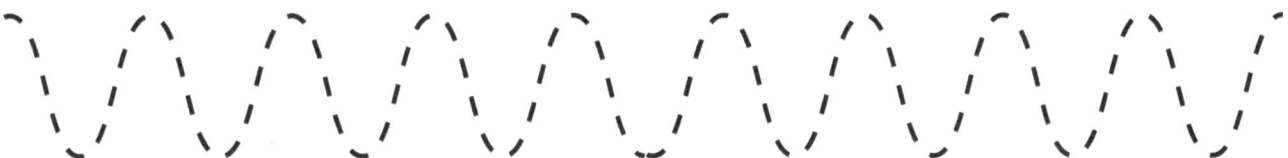

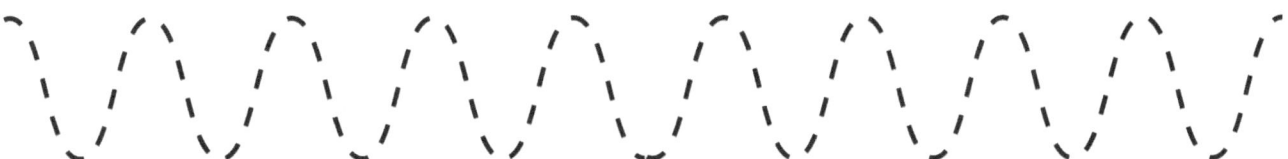

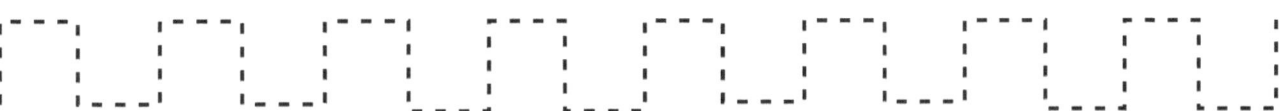

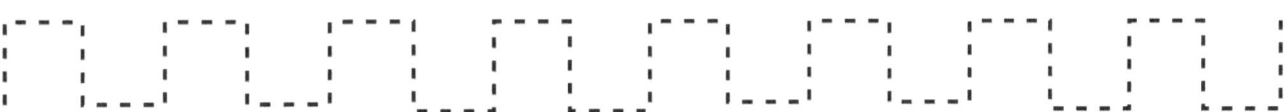

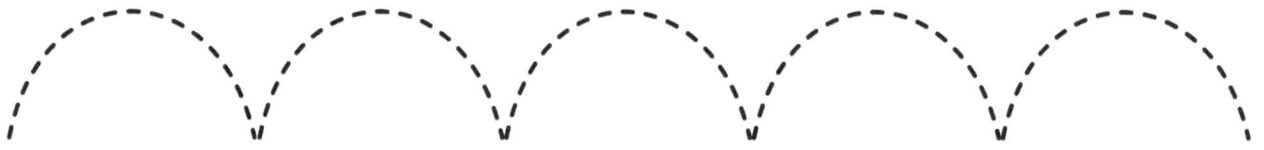

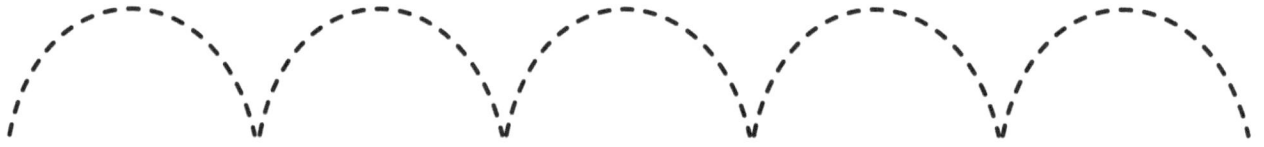

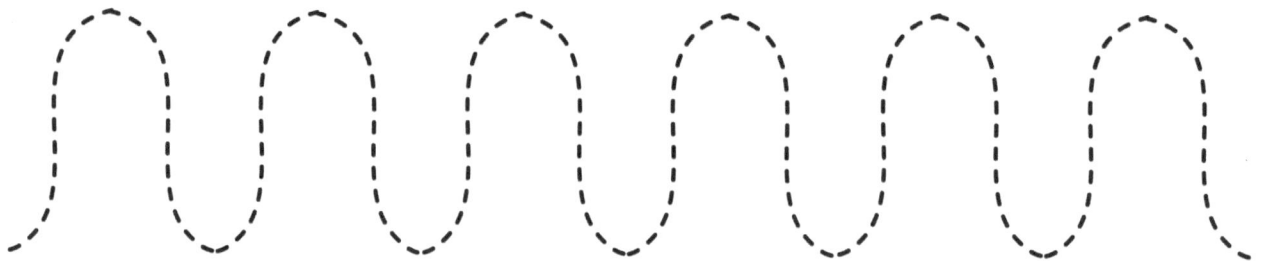

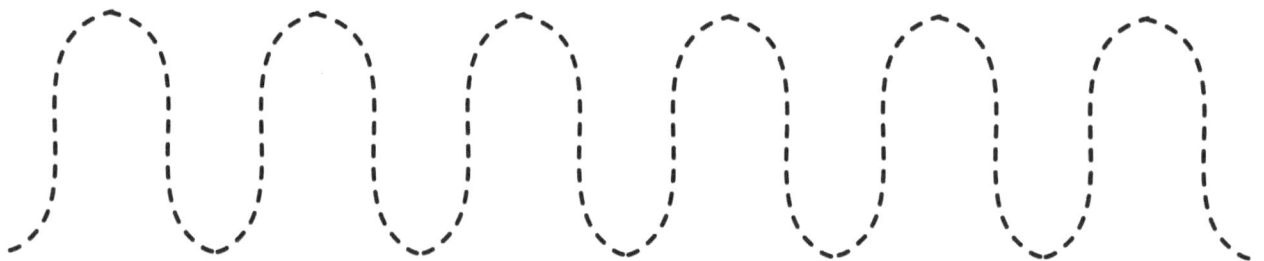

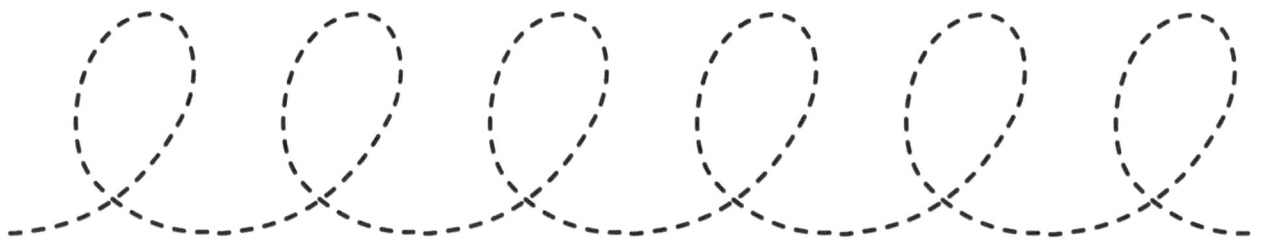

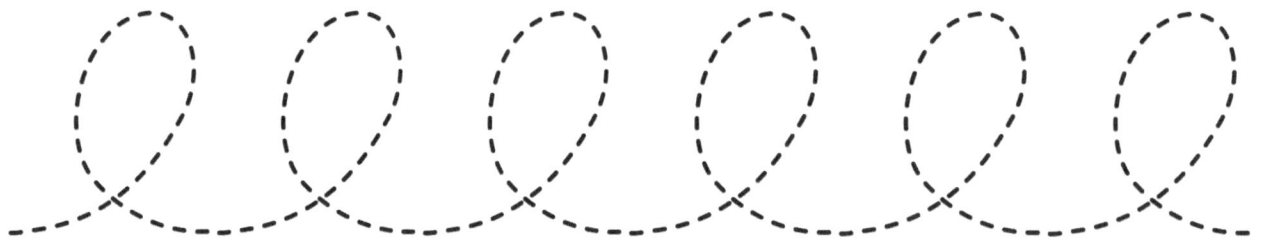

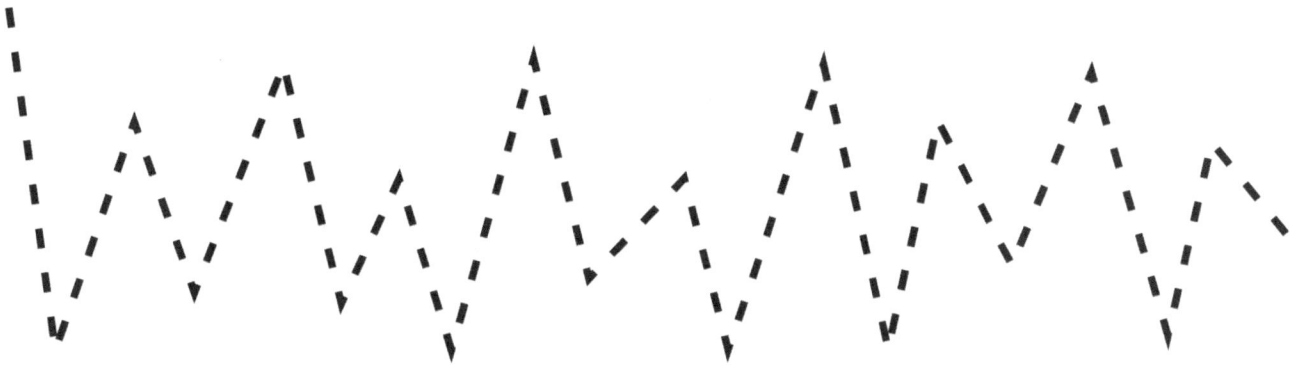

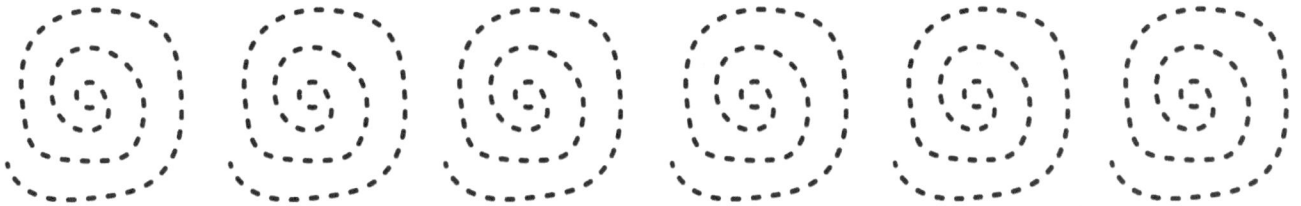

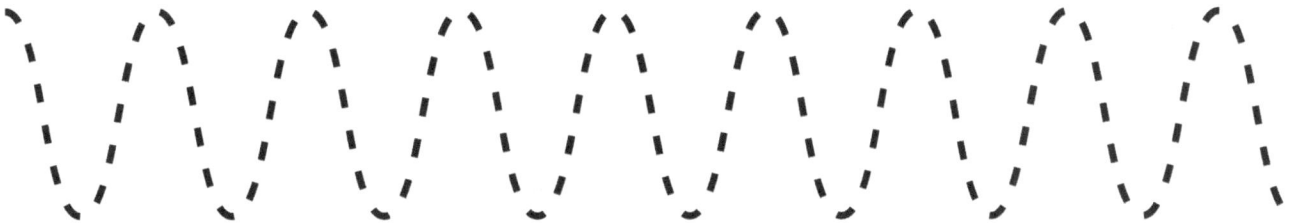

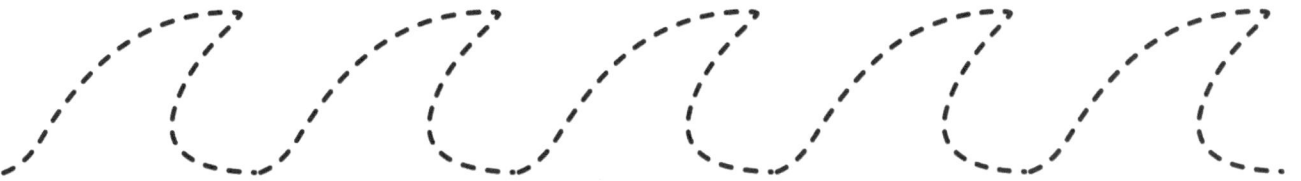

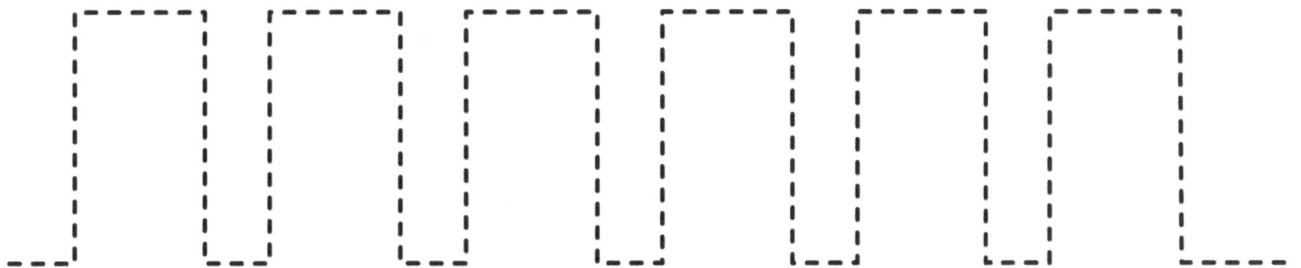

Read, trace, and color the shapes

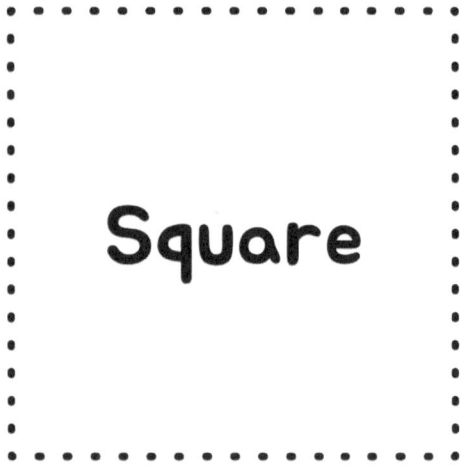

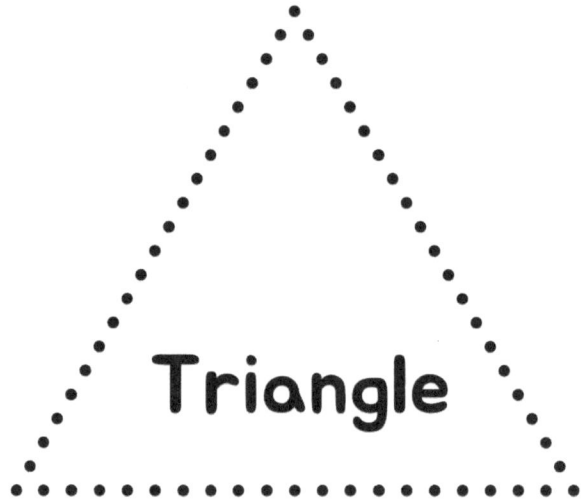

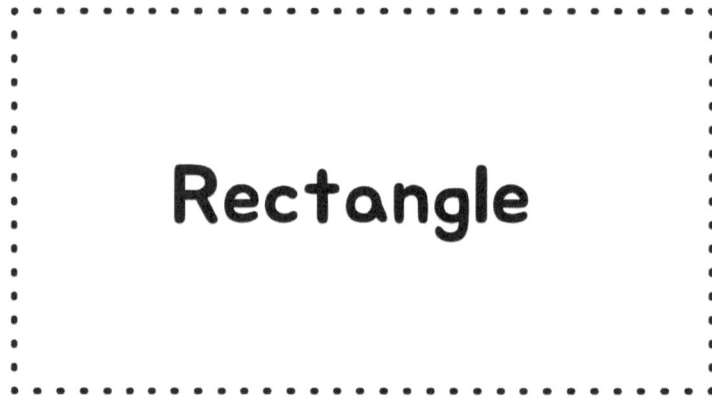

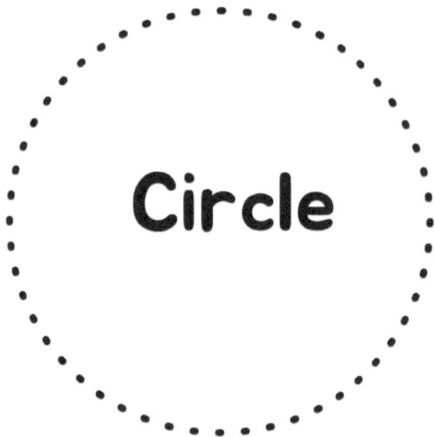

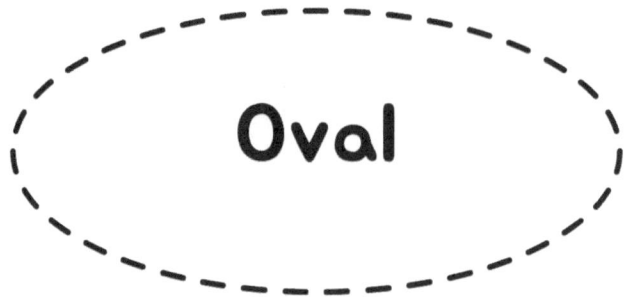

Square

Triangle

Rectangle

Circle

Oval

Trace and color the pictures

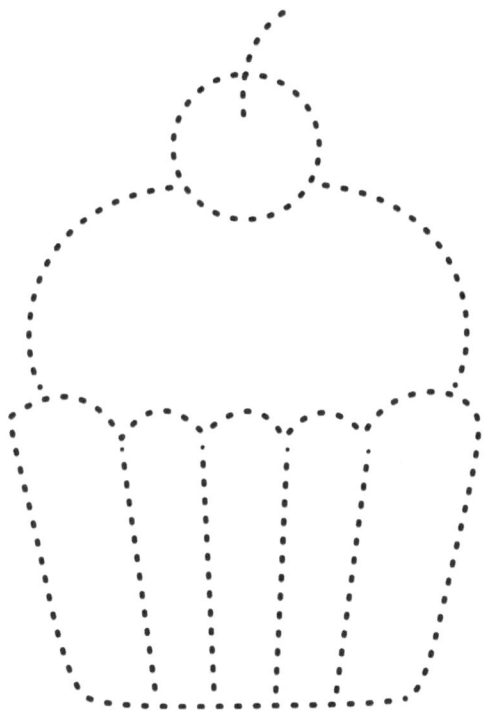

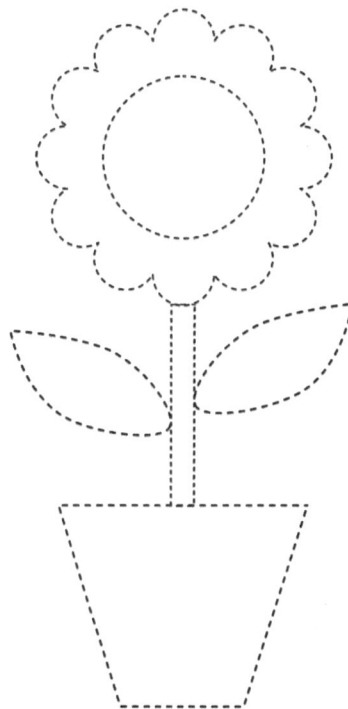

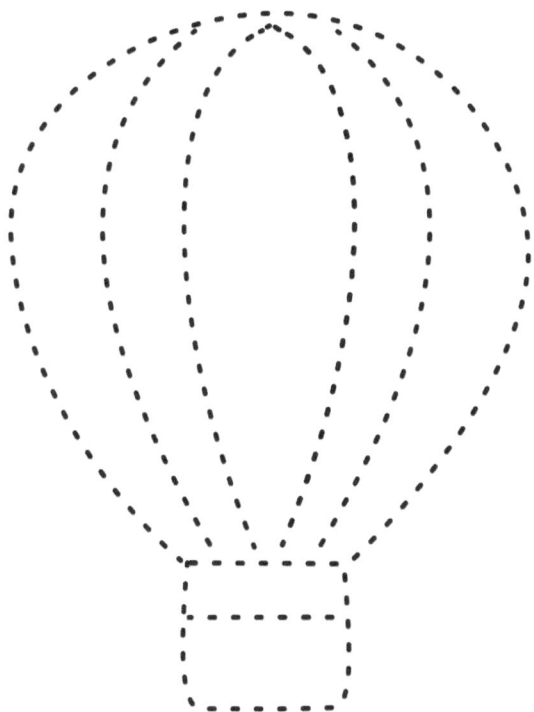

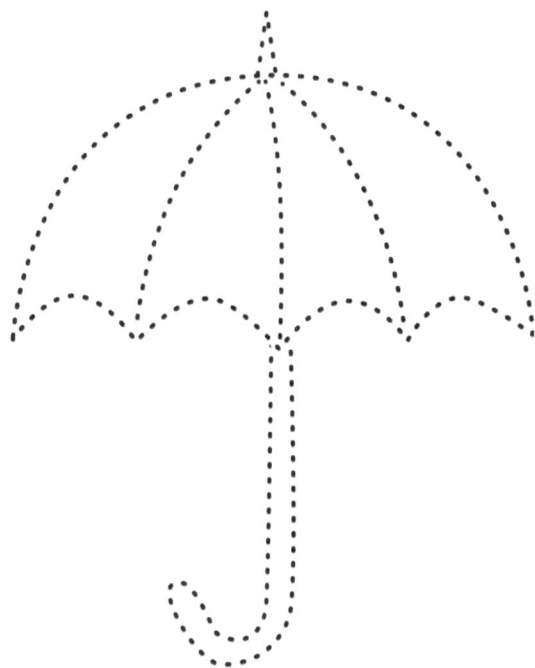

Trace the line following the dots

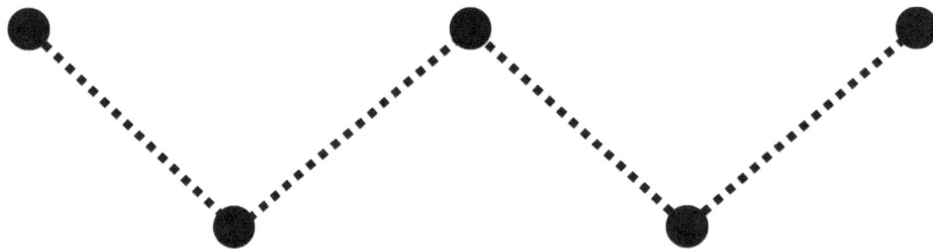

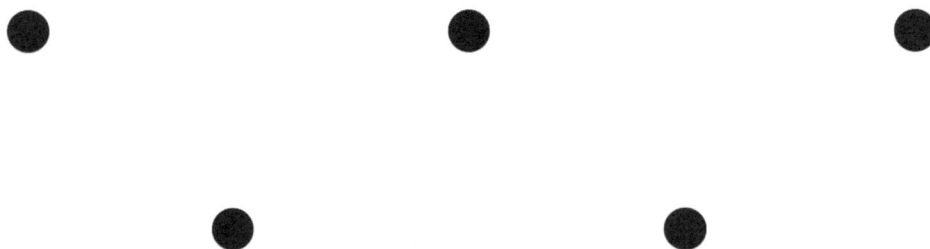

Trace the line following the dots

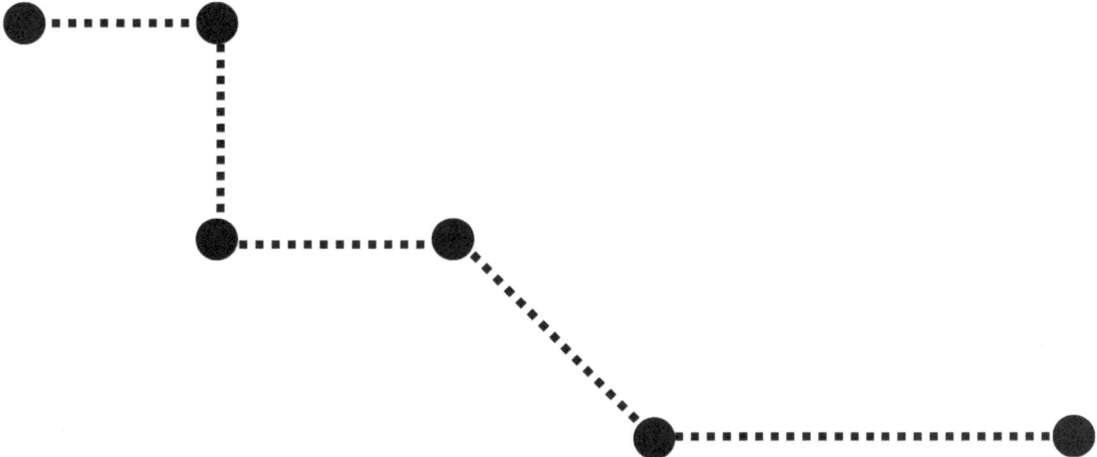

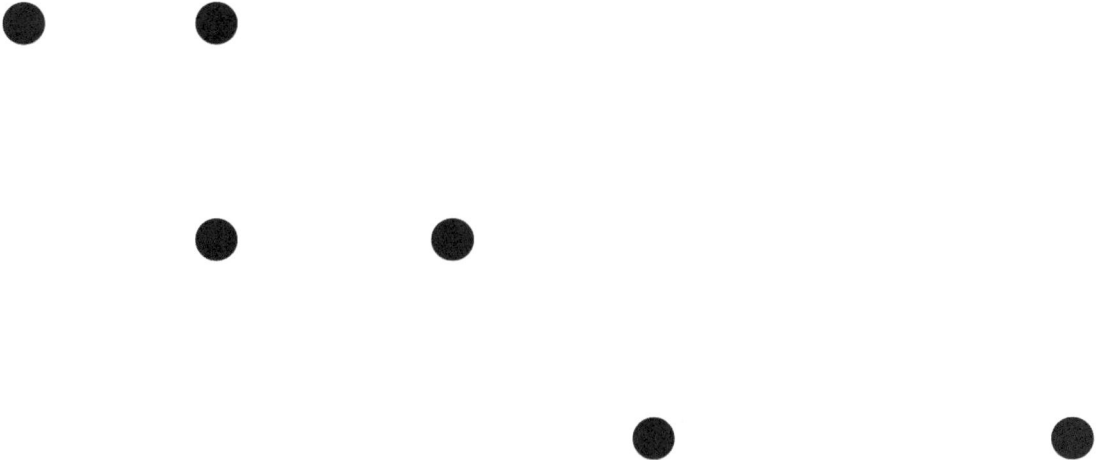

Trace the line following the dots

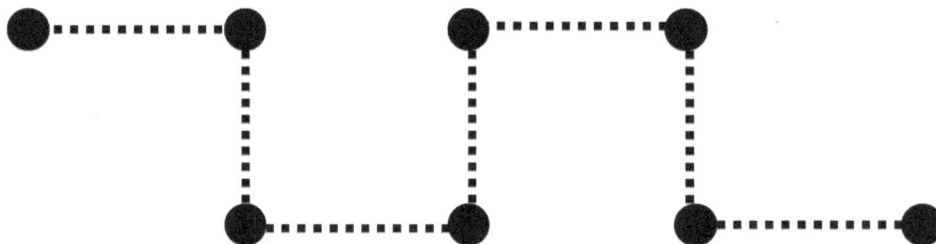

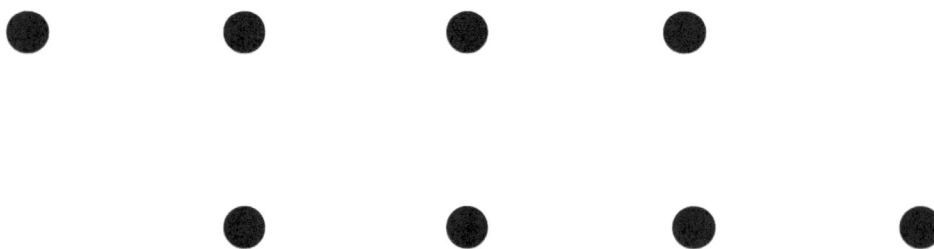

Trace the line following the dots

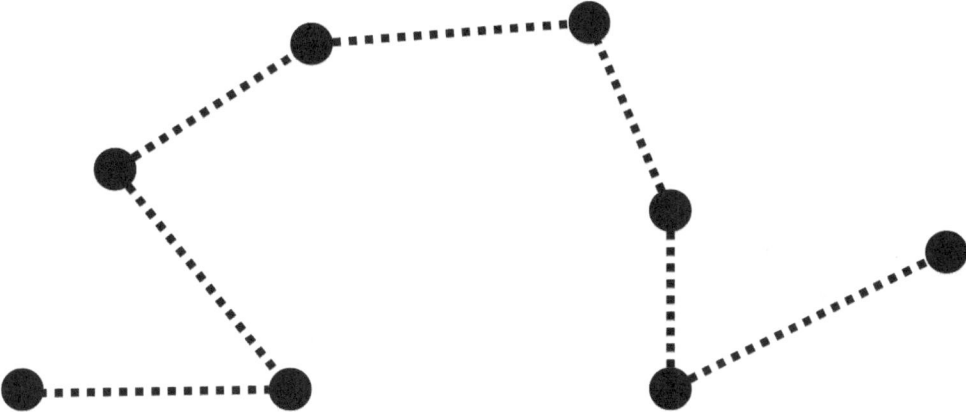

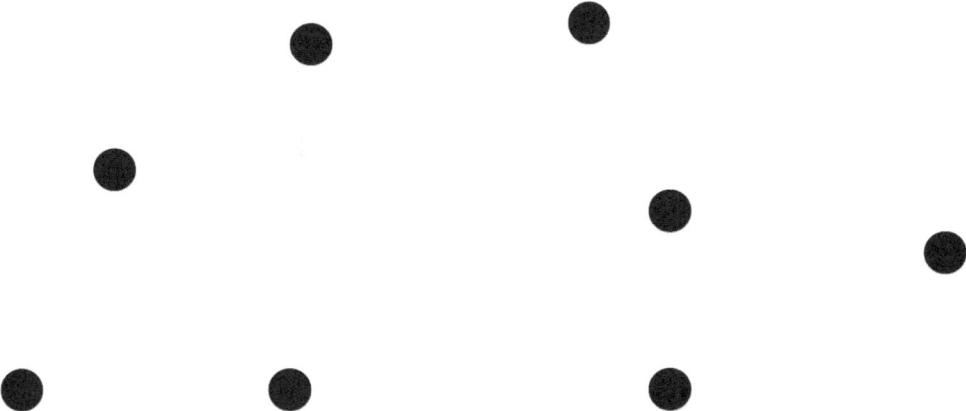

Trace the line following the dots

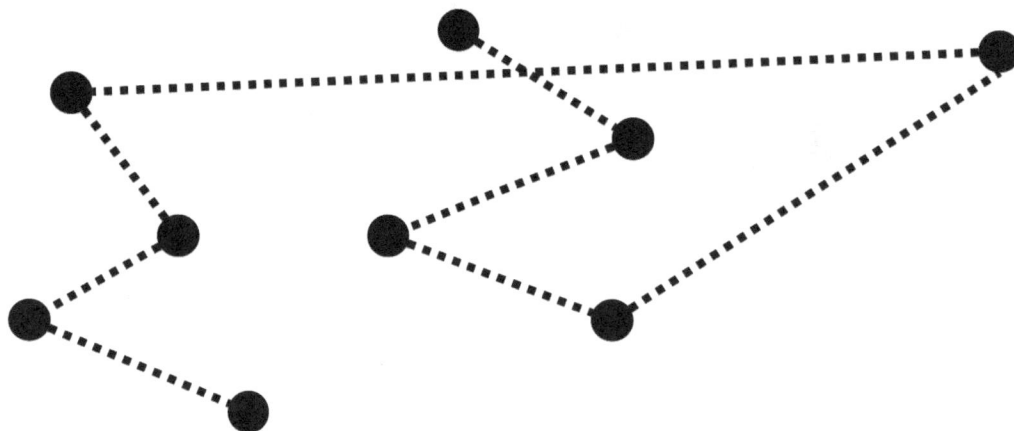

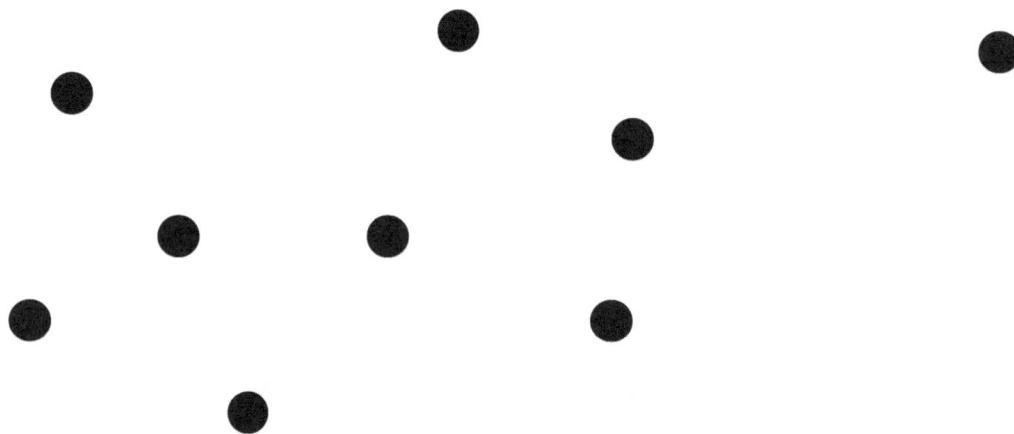

Trace and write the numbers

Aa Bb Cc Dd Ee

Ff Gg Hh Ii Jj Kk

Ll Mm Nn Oo Pp

Qq Rr Ss Tt Uu

Vv Ww Xx Yy Zz

1   5

2   6

3   7

4   8

Trace and write the days of the week

Pronounce them and choose which one is your favorite.

Monday

Tuesday

Wednesday

Thursday

Friday

Saturday

Sunday

Color, trace and draw the shapes

Color   Trace   Draw

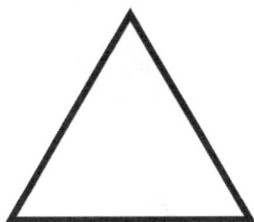 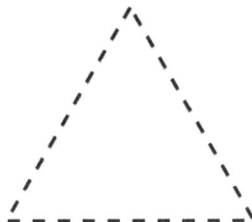 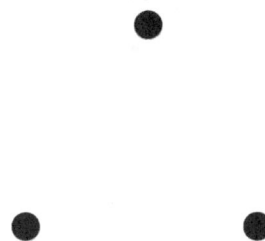

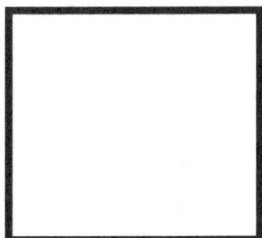  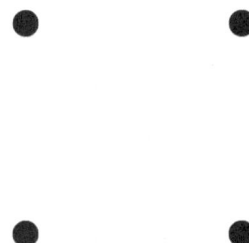

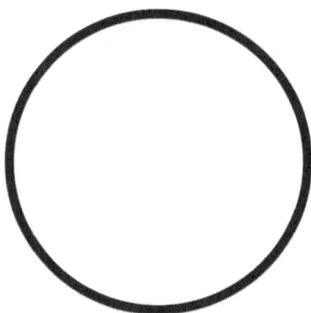  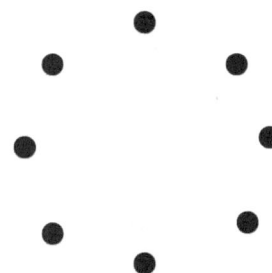

Symmetry

Match the two figures that show symmetry.

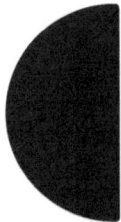

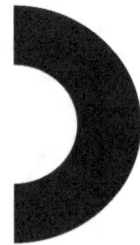

Mirror Image

Draw the other half of each shape.

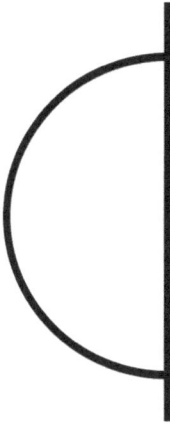

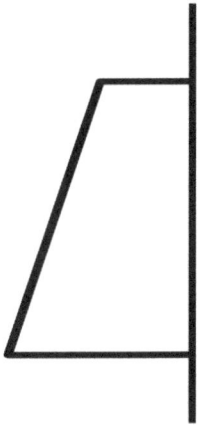

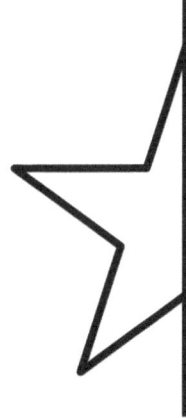

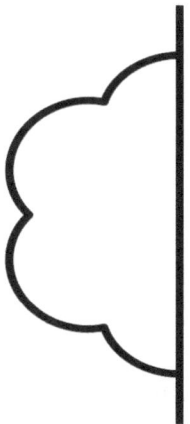

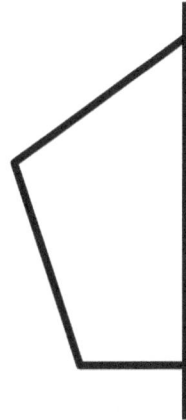

Symmetry

Complete these pictures by drawing the other half.

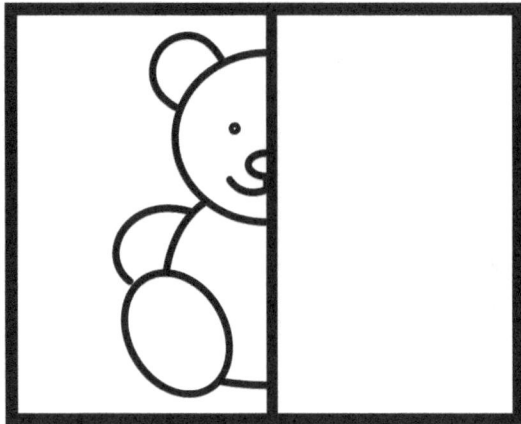

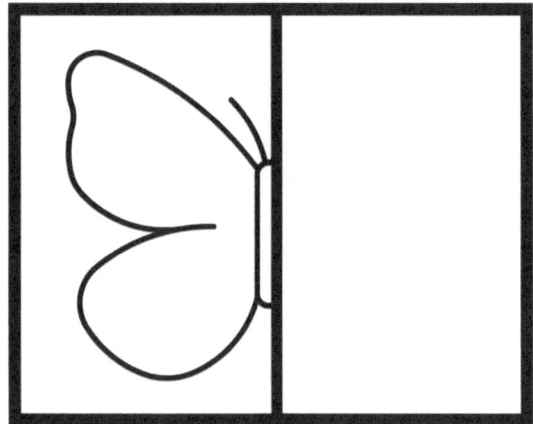

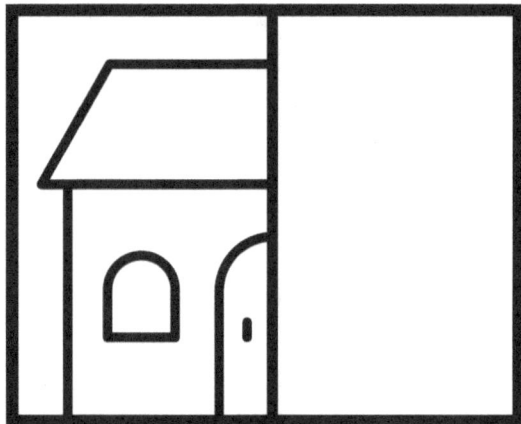

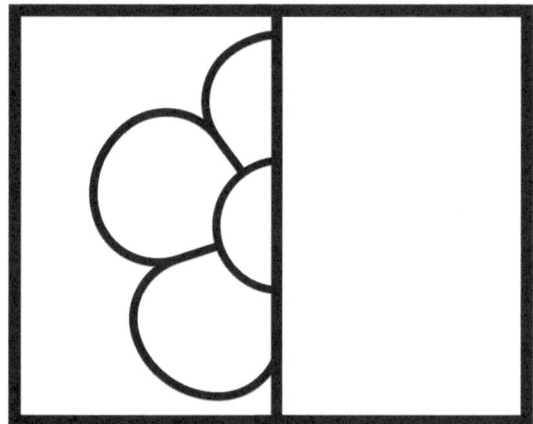

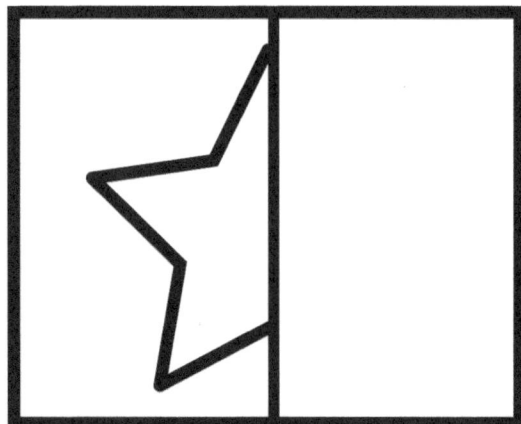

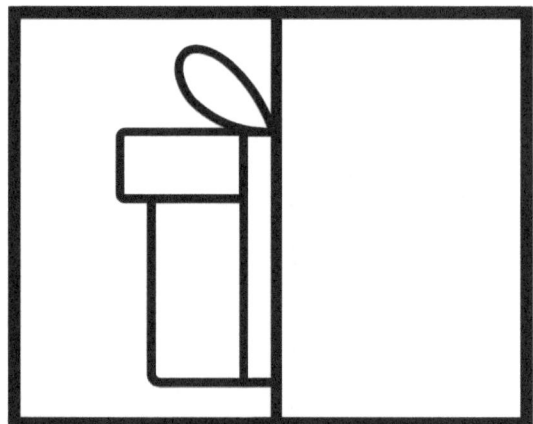

Trace and Draw your own

Color it.

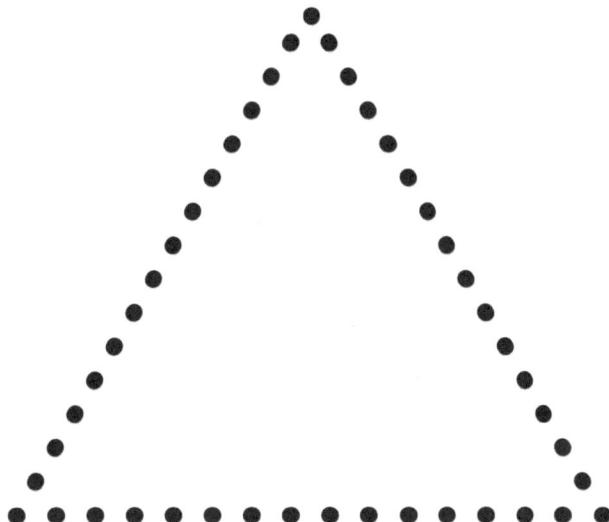

Trace and Draw your own

<u>Pronounce and write the name of the fruit.</u>

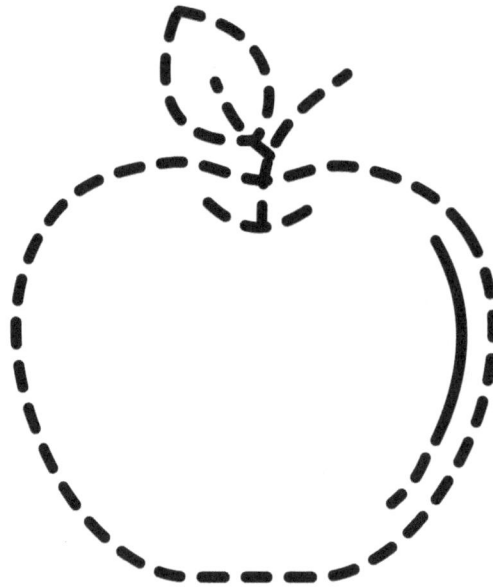

Trace and Draw your own

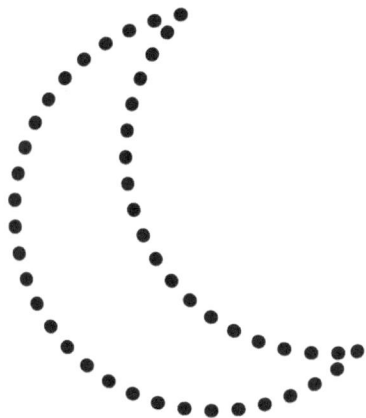

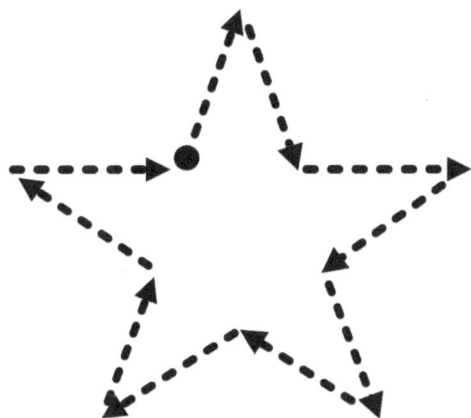

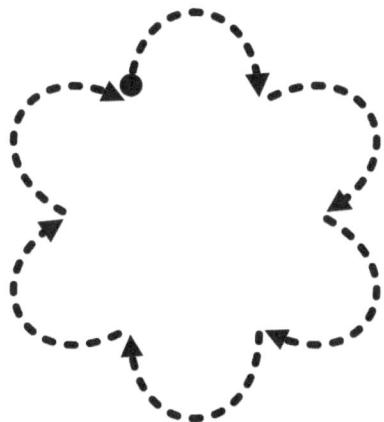

Trace and Draw your own

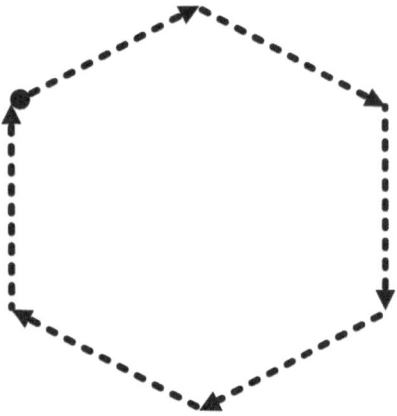

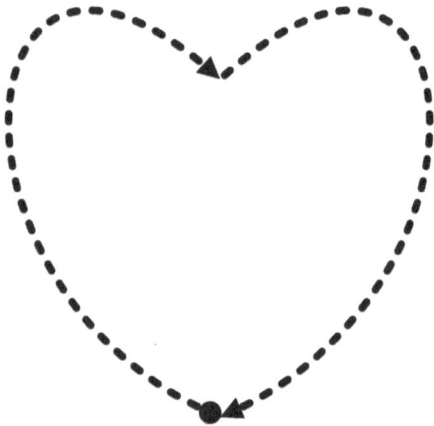

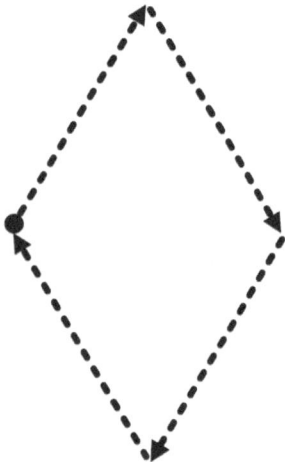

Trace and Draw your own

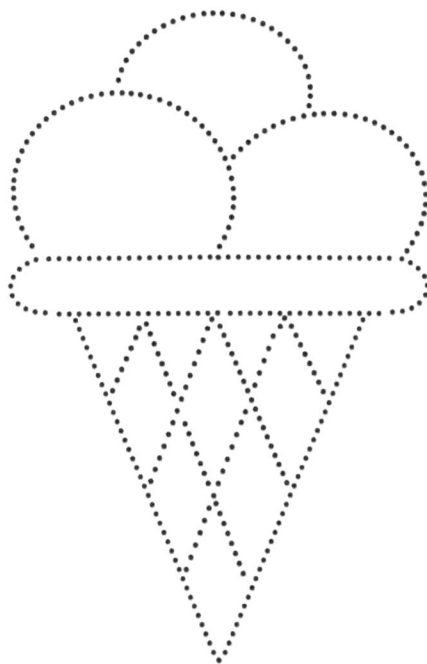

Trace and Draw your own

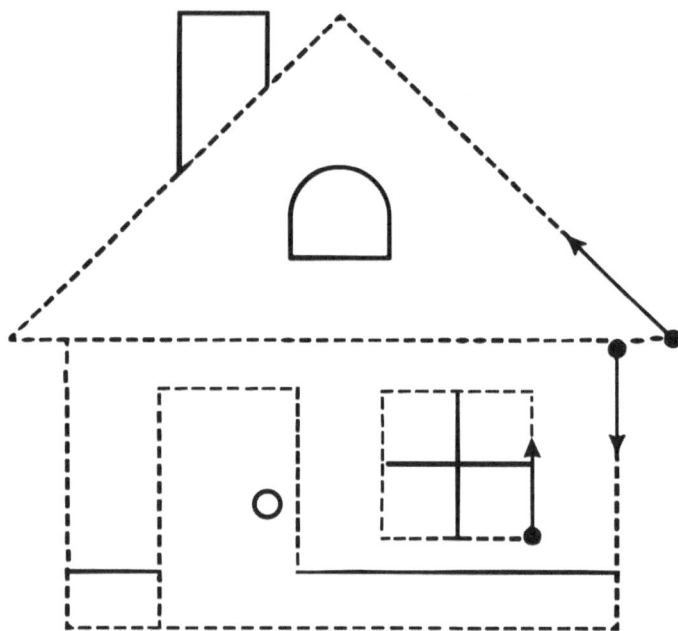

Emoji Game

Mime each emoji hand.

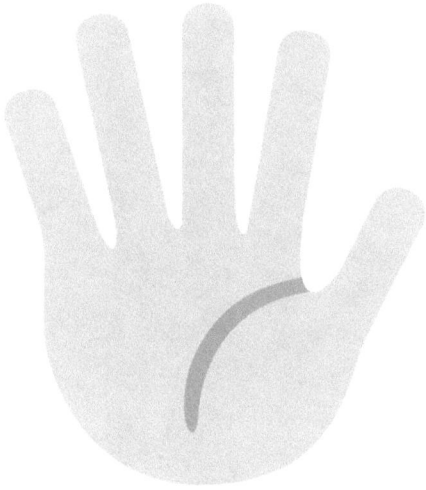

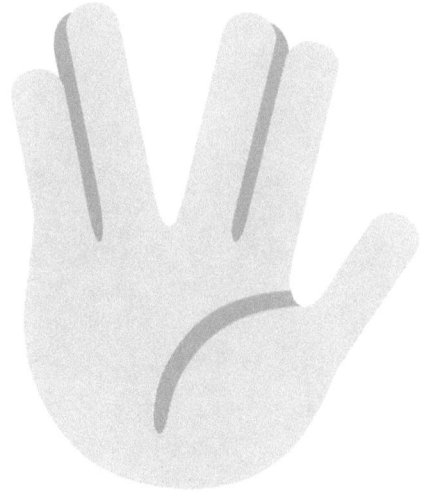

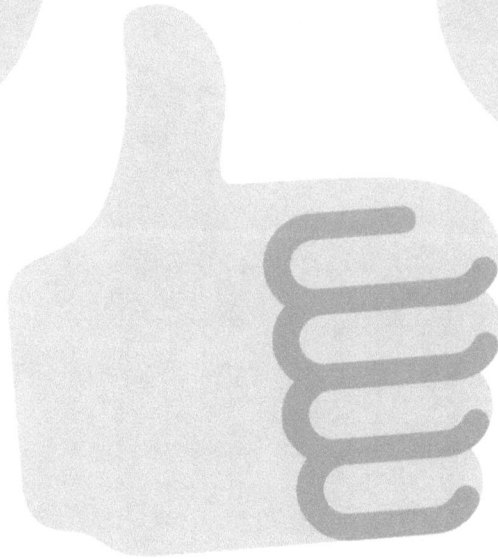

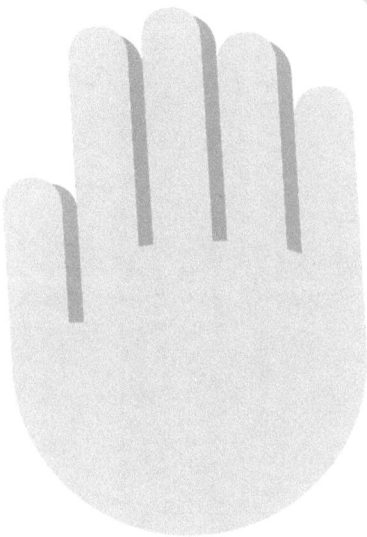

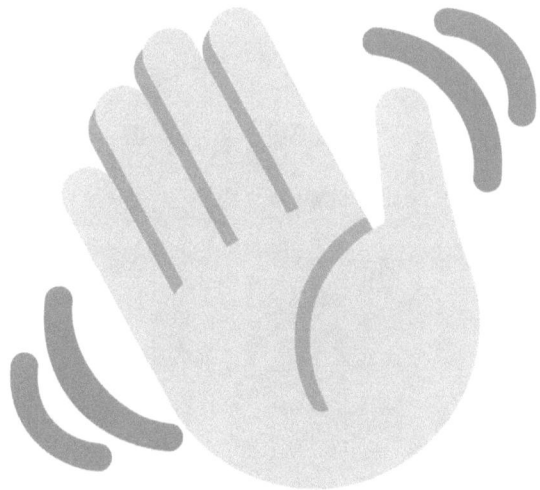

Emoji Game

Mime each emoji hand.

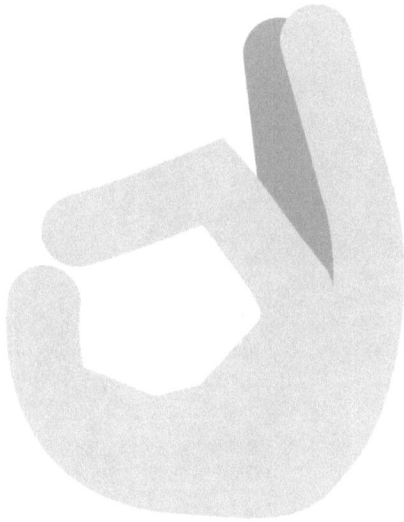

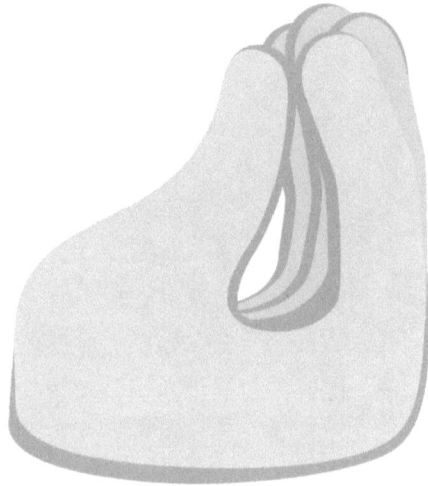

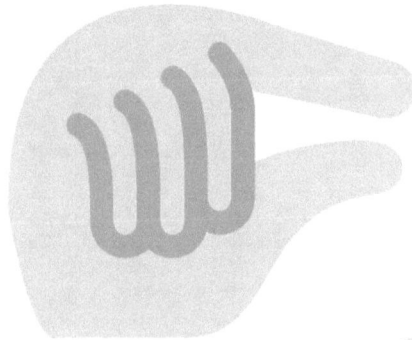

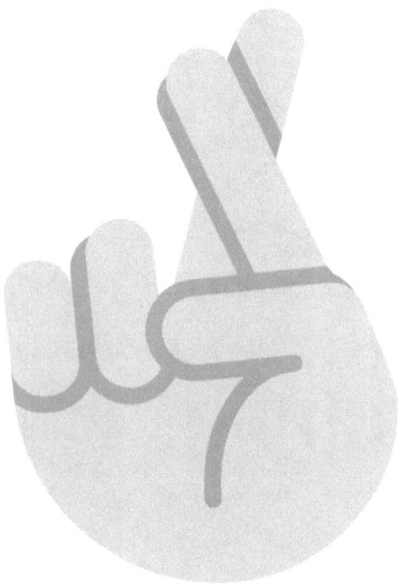

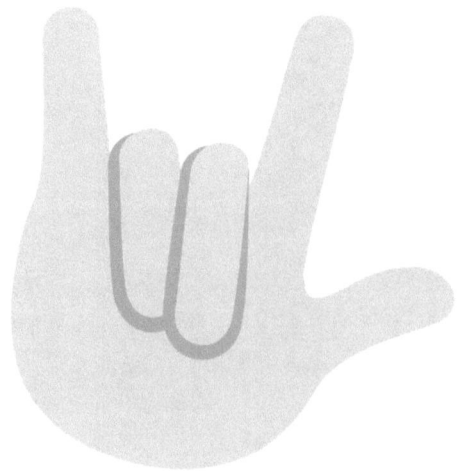

Emoji Game

Mime each emoji hand.

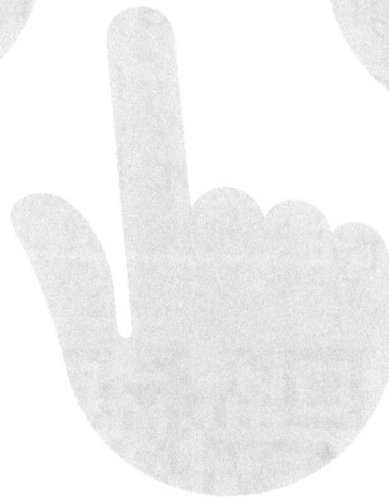

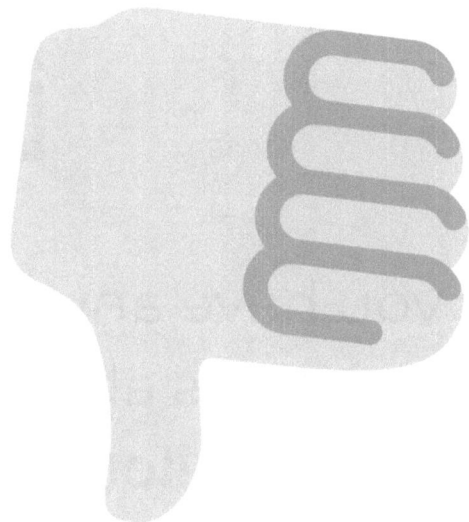

⭐⭐⭐⭐⭐

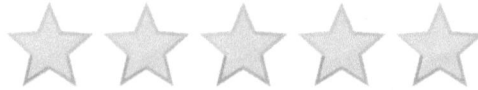

Enjoyed Your Experience? We'd Love to Hear From You!

Your feedback helps us grow and improve. If you enjoyed your experience with our book, please consider leaving a **review on Amazon**. It's a great way to support us and helps others benefit from what you've enjoyed. **Thank you** for being a crucial part of our community!

If you have any comments, suggestions or questions about this book, please email **hello@vitalstepsbooks.com**

Write down three things you are grateful for today and
how they made you feel.

_____

_____

_____

_____

_____

_____

_____

_____

_____

_____

_____

_____

_____

_____

_____

Write a letter to a friend explaining how your life has changed and what you have learned about yourself.

Describe your favorite place to relax and why it makes you feel at peace.

_____

_____

_____

_____

_____

_____

_____

_____

_____

_____

_____

_____

_____

_____

Write a short story about someone overcoming an obstacle. Use this narrative to reflect on your own challenges and victories.

Choose a goal for your rehabilitation. Describe the specific steps you will take to achieve this goal and why it is important to you.

_____

_____

_____

_____

_____

_____

_____

_____

_____

_____

_____

_____

_____

_____

Made in United States
Troutdale, OR
05/10/2024